THE CHAPTER <797> ANSWER BOOK

THE CHAPTER <797> ANSWER BOOK

2nd Edition

Patricia C. Kienle, RPh, MPA, BCSCP, FASHP

Director, Accreditation and Medication Safety

Cardinal Health

Any correspondence regarding this publication should be sent to the publisher, ASHP, 4500 East-West Highway, Suite 900, Bethesda, MD 20814, attention: Special Publishing.

The information presented herein reflects the opinions of the contributors and advisors. It should not be interpreted as an official policy of ASHP or as an endorsement of any product.

Because of ongoing research and improvements in technology, the information and its applications contained in this text are constantly evolving and are subject to the professional judgment and interpretation of the practitioner due to the uniqueness of a clinical situation. The editors and ASHP have made reasonable efforts to ensure the accuracy and appropriateness of the information presented in this document. However, any user of this information is advised that the editors and ASHP are not responsible for the continued currency of the information, for any errors or omissions, and/or for any consequences arising from the use of the information in the document in any and all practice settings. Any reader of this document is cautioned that ASHP makes no representation, guarantee, or warranty, express or implied, as to the accuracy and appropriateness of the information contained in this document and specifically disclaims any liability to any party for the accuracy and/or completeness of the material or for any damages arising out of the use or non-use of any of the information contained in this document.

Senior Vice President, Professional Development and Publishing Office: Daniel J. Cobaugh, PharmD, DABAT, FAACT

Editorial Director, Special Publishing: Ryan E. Owens, PharmD, BCPS

Director, Production and Platform Services, Publishing Operations: Johnna M. Hershey, BA

Production Services/Printing: Progressive Publishing Services/Sheridan

Cover Design: DeVall Advertising

Cover Art: iStock.com/beijingstory

Page Design: David Wade

Print ISBN: 978-1-58528-725-3

PDF ISBN: 978-1-58528-726-0

ePub ISBN: 978-1-58528-727-7

DOI: 10.37573/9781585287260

10 9 8 7 6 5 4 3 2 1

TABLE OF CONTENTS

DOI 10.37573/9781585287260.FM

PREFACE

The Chapter <797> Answer Book, 2nd edition, provides an explanation of elements of *USP <797> Sterile Preparations* and best practices to comply with the requirements and recommendations of the USP General Chapter.

The author is a member of the USP Compounding Expert Committee, but this publication is not endorsed by or affiliated with USP.

Comments in this book are related to USP chapters published as of November 1, 2022. The revised chapter is called the 2023 revision in this book. Revisions must be considered when designing policies and practices.

Patricia C. Kienle

Compounding IV Solutions in the 1930s

At that time [ca. 1930], [Dr. Harvey] Cushing's solution was formulated at each nursing unit by adding the contents of a powder pack, compounded individually in the hospital pharmacy, to a liter of boiling distilled water. After it cooled, the solution was poured into a burette and administered intravenously through used rubber tubing and a glass adapter affixed to a needle. The burette and tubing were sterilized by boiling in an instrument sterilizer. On wards that had a bedpan sterilizer, that was used. The glass burettes were stained and often opaque and sticky. In the operating room and in a cleaner context, nurse-anesthetists prepared and administered 5% dextrose in Cushing's solution, but reactions were masked by anesthesia.

— Walter CW. Finding a better way. *JAMA*. 1990; 263:1675-8.

INTRODUCTION

Information concerning compounding has been incorporated in the *United States Pharmacopeia* since the first publication in 1820. Specific guidance for sterile compounding is provided in *USP General Chapter <797> Pharmaceutical Compounding—Sterile Preparations* and has evolved as contemporary practice including:

- Originated as *USP General Chapter <1206> Sterile Drug Products for Home Use*
- First published as *USP General Chapter <797> Pharmaceutical Compounding—Sterile Preparations* in 2004
- Revised in 2008
- Published for public comment in 2015
- Public comments incorporated into second public comment version in 2018
- Proposed revision published in 2019, but was appealed
- Public comments (including discussion of appeals) incorporated into public comment version in 2021
- Revision published in 2022 with an extended one year official date of November 1, 2023[1]

Pharmacies and other entities where sterile compounding occurs should obtain a copy of the full document. It is available from the United States Pharmacopeial Convention (USP), either as a part of the full *USP–NF* (National Formulary), or as part of the *USP Compounding Compendium*.

The USP is recognized in the Federal Food, Drug, and Cosmetic Act as an official compendium.[2] ***Numbering of the chapters is significant:***

- USP chapters numbered below <1000> are considered applicable when they are referenced in a *General Notice*, a monograph, or in another general chapter numbered below <1000>.
- General Chapters numbered above <1000> are informational.
- Note that some regulatory agencies also consider those chapters above <1000> as requirements.

USP is a standard-setting organization, not a regulatory or enforcement agency. Regulatory bodies (such as the Centers for Medicare & Medicaid Services [CMS], state boards of pharmacy, state departments of health) and accreditation organizations enforce USP standards and/or include them in their standards.

In addition to USP <797>, other USP General Chapters also deal with compounding, including the following:

- *<795> Pharmaceutical Compounding—Nonsterile Preparations*
- *<800> Hazardous Drugs—Handling in Healthcare Settings*

DOI 10.37573/9781585287260.FM

- *<825> Radiopharmaceuticals—Preparation, Compounding, Dispensing, and Repackaging*
- *<1066> Physical Environments That Promote Safe Medication Use*
- *<1160> Pharmaceutical Calculations in Pharmacy Practice*
- *<1163> Quality Assurance in Pharmaceutical Compounding*
- *<1168> Compounding for Phase 1 Investigational Studies*
- *<1176> Prescription Balances and Volumetric Apparatus Used in Compounding*

Other USP General Chapters provide more specific information needed when certain types of compounded sterile preparations (CSPs) are mixed or to address compounding processes, including the following:

- *<7> Labeling*
- *<51> Antimicrobial Effectiveness Testing*
- *<71> Sterility Tests*
- *<85> Bacterial Endotoxins Test*
- *<659> Packaging and Storage Requirements*
- *<1085> Guidelines on Endotoxins Tests*
- *<1113> Microbial Characterization, Identification, and Strain Typing*
- *<1116> Microbial Control and Monitoring of Aseptic Processing Environments*
- *<1197> Good Distribution Practices for Bulk Pharmaceutical Excipients*
- *<1223> Validation of Alternative Microbial Methods*
- *<1228> Depyrogenation*
- *<1229> Sterilization of Compendial Articles*

References

1. United States Pharmacopeial Convention. General chapter <797> hazardous drugs—handling in healthcare settings. *USP-NF 2023*, Issue 1, November 1, 2022.

2. United States Code, Title 21, §321, http://uscode.house.gov/view.xhtml?req=%28official+compendium%29+AND+%28%28title%3A%2821%29%29%29&f=treesort&fq=true&num=0&hl=true&edition=prelim&granuleId=USC-prelim-title21--section321. Accessed November 1, 2022.

ACKNOWLEDGMENTS

Current and past members of the USP Compounding Expert Committee devoted countless volunteer hours to research, discussion, and development of practices to help ensure patient safety. Many thanks to them, to Kate Douglass, and to USP staff Richard Schnatz, Jeanne Sun, Tiffany Chan, Abbey Ammerman, Brian Serumaga, and Selma Mitiche.

REVIEWERS

Brenda Jensen, CPhT, CNMT, MBA

Pharmacy Consultant
Compounding Consultants, LLC
Sioux Falls, South Dakota

Michael J. Winstanley, RPh, BCSCP

Sterile Compounding Supervisor
Jersey Shore University Medical Center
Neptune, New Jersey

ACD	automated compounding device
ACPH	air changes per hour
ACS	American Chemical Society
AECA	allergenic extracts compounding area
API	active pharmaceutical ingredient
APIC	Association for Professionals in Infection Control and Epidemiology
ASHP	American Society of Health-System Pharmacists
ASTM	American Society for Testing and Materials
BPS	Board of Pharmacy Specialties
BSC	biological safety cabinet
BUD	beyond-use date
C-SCA	containment segregated compounding area
CACI	compounding aseptic containment isolator
CAG	certification application guide
CAI	compounding aseptic isolator
CDC	Centers for Disease Control and Prevention
CETA	Controlled Environment Testing Association
CFU	colony-forming unit
CNBT	CETA National Board of Testing
CoA	certificate of analysis
CR	compounding record
CSP	compounded sterile preparation
CVE	containment ventilated enclosure
EM	environmental monitoring
FD&C Act	Food, Drug, & Cosmetic Act
FDA	U.S. Food and Drug Administration
HD	hazardous drug
HEPA	high-efficiency particulate air
ISO	International Standards Organization
LTC	long-term care
MEA	malt extract agar
MFR	master formulation record
NF	National Formulary
NIOSH	National Institute for Occupational Safety and Health
NRC	Nuclear Regulatory Commission
OSHA	Occupational Safety and Health Administration
PBP	pharmacy bulk package
PEC	primary engineering control
PNSU	probability of nonsterile unit
PPE	personal protective equipment
PTCB	Pharmacy Technician Certification Board
QA	quality assurance

DOI 10.37573/9781585287260.FM

ACRONYMS (continued)

QC	quality control
RABS	restricted-access barrier system
RAM License	radioactive materials license
SCA	segregated compounding area
SDA	Sabouraud dextrose agar
SDS	safety data sheet; formerly called material safety data sheet (MSDS)
SEC	secondary engineering control
sIPA	sterile 70% isopropyl alcohol
SOP	standard operating procedure
SRPA	segregated radiopharmaceutical processing area
TPN	total parenteral nutrition
TSA	trypticase soy agar
USP	United States Pharmacopeial Convention *United States Pharmacopeia*
wc	water column

Unless otherwise noted, compounding discussed in this text refers to nonhazardous sterile compounding.

DISCLAIMER

This book is based on the revision of USP <797> that was published on November 1, 2022 and is official as of November 1, 2023. The 2008 version of USP <797> remains in effect through October 31, 2023.

The 2023 revision of USP <797> expanded explanatory information and updated many requirements. The following chart provides an overview of the major changes:

Topic	2008 Version	2023 Revision
Risk categories	Low, medium, and high	Elimination of this distinction
Categories of compounded sterile preparations (CSPs)		Categories 1, 2, and 3 are based on the facility in which a CSP is compounded and, for Category 3, if beyond use dates (BUDs) are extended beyond those allowed for Category 2
Immediate use	Maximum BUD of 1 hour.	Maximum BUD of 4 hours.
	Maximum of 3 sterile components and 2 entries into any one container.	Maximum of 3 different sterile products.
Administration	Administration and preparation per manufacturer's labeling included in description of compounding	Administration and preparation per manufacturer's labeling is out of scope of <797> as long as it is intended for a single patient and will not be stored
Personnel		Requirement for designated person
Personnel monitoring frequency	Every 12 months for low- and medium-risk; every 6 months for high-risk	Every 6 months for Category 1 and 2, and every 3 months for Category 3. Annually for some other personnel (see text).
		Addition of surface sampling following media fill and gloved fingertip sampling
Facility design	Allowance for placement of containment primary engineering controls (C-PECs) outside of negative pressure if only a low volume of hazardous drugs (HDs) compounded	Elimination of this exemption, because all HD compounding (unless exempted in the Assessment of Risk) must occur in negative pressure room
	Sink placement on clean side of anteroom	Sink placement based on facility design and work practices
Placement of compounding aseptic isolator (CAI) outside of cleanroom suite	Allowance for full beyond-use dates (BUDs)	Full BUDs can only be assigned if the CAI is placed in a cleanroom suite
BUDs in a segregated compounding area (SCA)	Maximum of 12 hours	Maximum of 12 hours room temperature or 24 hours refrigerated
BUDs	See details in chapter	See details in chapter, including limitations
Documentation		Master formulation records and compounding records required
Facility surface sampling	Required periodically	Required monthly

DOI 10.37573/9781585287260.FM

LIST OF QUESTIONS

Answers to questions marked "revised" have been updated since the first edition of this book.

Chapter 1: USP <797> Availability

1.1	Where can I find the full text of <797>?
1.2 REVISED	When did <797> become official?
1.3	Why is there a need for a chapter on sterile compounding? Is this all about the meningitis scare from 2012?
1.4	Is <797> a guideline? A requirement?
1.5	How can <797> be a minimum standard if my state hasn't incorporated it into regulations?

Chapter 2: General Principles of USP <797>

2.1	Is USP <797> a new chapter?
2.2 REVISED	What is the status of the proposed revisions published between 2008 and 2021?
2.3	When must I comply with <797>?
2.4	What is the distinction between the terms *must* and *should* in the text of <797>?
2.5	If I'm just repackaging sterile products into unit doses, do I need to comply with <797>?
2.6	Are hazardous drugs addressed in <797>?
2.7	Are radiopharmaceuticals addressed in <797>?
2.8	Are allergens addressed in <797>?

Chapter 3: Contents of Sections of USP <797>

No questions

Chapter 4: Scope of USP <797>

4.1	Who has to comply with <797>?
4.2	I've heard <797> referred to as a guideline and a standard. Which is correct? What's the difference?
4.3	Is <797> a regulation?
4.4	Does <797> apply to animals?
4.5	Can I select certain sections of <797> to be compliant with?
4.6 REVISED	Is <797> in effect now?
4.7 REVISED	What are examples of preparations that must comply—and those that do not comply—with <797>?
4.8	Does <797> apply to all compounds?
4.9	Does <797> apply to investigational agents?
4.10 REVISED	I work in a hospital pharmacy. Do I need to comply with <795> or <797>?
4.11	Does <800> replace <797>?
4.12	Do community or mail-order pharmacies have to comply with <797>? How about a private physician's office?
4.13	Do pharmaceutical manufacturers have to comply with <797>?
4.14	Does a nursing home have to comply with <797>?
4.15 REVISED	What types of activities aren't considered compounding?
4.16 REVISED	How is administering medications distinguished from compounding?
4.17 REVISED	What is the time limit for Immediate Use?
4.18	Does <797> include prepackaging from a vial to a unit-dose syringe?
4.19	<795> says repackaging is out of scope. Why is it included in <797>?
4.20	Is it OK to compound a preparation that can be mixed cheaper than the commercial product?
4.21	Who will enforce <797> for compliance outside of pharmacy settings?

LIST OF QUESTIONS (continued)

7.1-5	Is additional garb required for personnel who are compounding from powders?
7.1-6 REVISED	Do I need to wear garb if the hood I work in is a glove box?
7.1-7	What does *donning* and *doffing* mean?
7.1-8	Does the pharmacist who is only checking items need to garb?
7.1-9 REVISED	Can garb be reused?
7.1-10	The pharmacists and technicians who work in our operating room (OR) satellite wear "OR greens." Is this sufficient garb?
7.2	**HAND HYGIENE**
7.2-1	What does *hand hygiene* mean?
7.2-2	Can alcohol-based hand rub be used instead of soap and water?
7.2-3	How long should our policy say to wash hands?
7.2-4	Are regular paper towels OK to use?
7.3	**GLOVES**
7.3-1	When gloves are mentioned in <797>, what kind of gloves does that mean?
7.3-2	Is it OK to wash gloves between compounds?
7.3-3	When are sterile gloves required?
7.3-4	We use gloves boxes so put on gloves outside of the glove box. Is this correct?
7.3-5 REVISED	Are sterile gloves required when working in a compounding isolator?
7.3-6 REVISED	How often do compounding isolator gloves need to be changed?
7.3-7	Do chemo gloves have to meet a particular standard?
7.3-8	How do I know if a glove is chemo-rated?
7.3-9	Is it OK for chemo gloves to be tested per ASTM D6978 and laboratory chemical tested per ASTM F739?
7.4	**GOWNS**
7.4-1 REVISED	Do gowns have to be sterile?
7.4-2	What is the difference between gowns we use for non-HDs and those used for chemo?
7.4-3 REVISED	Can I hang my gown in the anteroom for use later in the day?
7.4-4 REVISED	Are washable gowns OK to use?
7.4-5	Do I need to wear a regular gown under my chemo gown?
7.5	**HAIR COVERS**
7.5-1	What is the difference between head and beard covers used for chemo and those used for nonhazardous CSPs?
7.5-2	One of our employees is completely bald. Does he need to wear a hair cover?
7.5-3	If personnel wear a head cover for religious or other reasons, is an additional hair cover necessary?
7.5-4	Do earrings have to be removed, or can they just be covered by the hair cover?
7.6	**MASKS**
7.6-1	Do I have to wear a surgical mask when compounding?
7.6-2	Is a mask the same thing as a respirator?
7.6-3	Is a face shield a mask?
7.7	**SLEEVES**
7.7-1	Are sleeve covers required?
7.8	**SHOE COVERS**
7.8-1	What is the difference between shoe covers used for chemo and those used for non-HDs?
7.8-2 REVISED	Can I use dedicated cleanroom shoes instead of shoe covers?

LIST OF QUESTIONS (continued)

Chapter 8: Immediate Use and Preparation for Administration

LIST OF QUESTIONS (continued)

LIST OF QUESTIONS (continued)

9.4-7	Can a person garb once and use three sets of plates at one time for the initial gloved fingertip and thumb test?
9.4-8	Do the three separate garbing sessions need to be done on the same day?
9.4-9 REVISED	How and where is the requalification gloved fingertip and thumb test done?
9.4-10	We use a compounding aseptic isolator (CAI). Does the gloved fingertip and thumb test need to be done inside the CAI?
9.4-11 REVISED	How often is the requalification gloved fingertip and thumb test required?
9.4-12 REVISED	Are three sets of media plates required for the requalification gloved fingertip and thumb test?
9.4-13	If someone passes two of the initial three gloved fingertip and thumb tests, do they have to repeat all three or just one?
9.4-14 REVISED	Is the training gloved fingertip and thumb test different from the one for requalification?
9.4-15	What does the *action level* mean?
9.4-16	Do the action level numbers apply to one hand or both hands?
9.4-17	Do you need to sample both hands?
9.4-18	Can one plate be used for both hands?
9.4-19 REVISED	What is the action level for the initial gloved fingertip and thumb test?
9.4-20 REVISED	What is the action level for the requalification gloved fingertip and thumb test?
9.4-21 REVISED	Why must I have no growth on a gloved fingertip and thumb test when I'm learning, but when I'm really mixing IVs for patients, I can have some growth?
9.4-22 REVISED	If someone exceeds the action level, are they allowed to compound?
9.4-23	Do nurses who only mix immediate-use CSPs need to do a gloved fingertip and thumb test?
9.4-24	Do the nuclear medicine technologists need to do a gloved fingertip and thumb test?
9.4-25 NEW	What is the purpose of surface sampling during personnel evaluation?
9.5	**ASEPTIC TECHNIQUE**
9.5-1	What is the definition of *aseptic technique*?
9.5-2	Is there a USP chapter about aseptic technique?
9.5-3	Does ASHP have any resources to teach aseptic technique?
9.5-4	Is the aseptic technique nurses learn or the technique used in the operating room (OR) the same thing as the aseptic technique we need to use when compounding?
9.5-5 REVISED	What test is used to demonstrate competence in aseptic technique?
9.6	**MEDIA FILL TEST**
9.6-1	What is the purpose of the media fill test?
9.6-2 REVISED	How often does a media fill test have to be done?
9.6-3	How do I design a media fill test?
9.6-4	Can I use a commercially available kit for a media fill test?
9.6-5	What kind of media and devices are used for a media fill test?
9.6-6	We use a CAI. Do we still need to do a media fill test?
9.6-7	Does everyone on staff need to do the same media fill test?
9.6-8	What is the proper procedure for doing a media fill test?
9.6-9	If I mix nonsterile-to-sterile preparations, can I use purchased soybean-casein digest media?
9.6-10	Can I start with nonsterile media and mix it myself?
9.6-11	Is there specific information I need to keep concerning the media used?
9.6-12 REVISED	Do I need an incubator?
9.6-13	Can I use a mannitol warmer to incubate the media fill tests?
9.6-14	At what temperature and for how long do the media fill tests need to be incubated?

LIST OF QUESTIONS (continued)

LIST OF QUESTIONS (continued)

LIST OF QUESTIONS (continued)

LIST OF QUESTIONS (continued)

11.7-3 REVISED	I have a combined ante/buffer room. Is this a cleanroom suite?
11.7-4	What is the ISO requirement for a cleanroom suite?
11.7-5	Are ceiling HEPA filters required?
11.7-6	I have HEPA filters in the ceiling and the air returns about a foot down from the ceiling. Is this OK?
11.7-7	Does a cleanroom suite require an isolator?
11.7-8 REVISED	I have a combined anteroom/buffer room that is ISO 7. I heard this is no longer allowed in new <797>. Is this true?
11.7-9 REVISED	Where does the sink need to be placed in a cleanroom suite?
11.7-10	Are there separate requirements for a cleanroom suite used for chemo?
11.7-11	Can the air conditioning be turned off in the cleanroom suite when it's not in use?
11.7-12	Can the number of air changes per hour be lowered when the cleanroom suite is not in use?
11.7-13	Are portable HEPA filters OK to use?
11.7-14	How many people can work in a cleanroom suite?
11.8	SEGREGATED COMPOUNDING AREAS FOR NONHAZARDOUS CSPs
11.8-1	What are the minimum room requirements for an SCA?
11.8-2	What can be mixed in an SCA?
11.8-3	Can all CSPs be mixed in an SCA?
11.8-4	What does a cleanroom suite have that an SCA doesn't have?
11.8-5	What is the purpose of a perimeter around the hood?
11.8-6 REVISED	Where does the sink need to be placed in an SCA?
11.8-7	Are there separate requirements for an SCA used for chemo?
11.8-8	What is the ISO requirement for an SCA?
11.9	CONTAINMENT SEGREGATED COMPOUNDING AREAS FOR HAZARDOUS CSPs
11.9-1	What are the minimum room requirements for a C-SCA?
11.9-2	Can I use a C-SCA for mixing all CSPs—both hazardous and not?
11.9-3	What does a cleanroom suite have that a C-SCA doesn't have?
11.9-4	Where does the sink need to be placed in a C-SCA?
11.9-5	What is the ISO requirement for a C-SCA?
11.10	PASS-THROUGH CHAMBERS
11.10-1	What is a pass-through?
11.10-2	What components make a pass-through cleanroom-compliant?
11.10-3	How big can a pass-through chamber be?
11.10-4 REVISED	Can a pass-through go from unclassified space into a cleanroom?
11.10-5	What testing is needed for a pass-through chamber?
11.10-6	How can I tell if the pass-through is contributing to problems in the IV room?
11.10-7	We have a window that slides open between the anteroom and buffer room. Is this a pass-through chamber?
11.10-8	Is a window OK in the pass-through chamber?
11.10-9 REVISED	Does the pass-through chamber need to be HEPA-filtered?
11.10-10	I have a HEPA-filtered pass-through. Can I turn off the HEPA filter when it's not in use?
11.10-11	Do HEPA-filtered pass-throughs need to be ISO classified?
11.10-12	How big are pass-through chambers?
11.10-13	Is it OK to pass supplies through a pass-through?
11.10-14	Our pass-through isn't interlocked, but we only allow opening one side at a time. Is this OK?

LIST OF QUESTIONS (continued)

LIST OF QUESTIONS (continued)

Chapter 12: Daily Nonviable Monitoring

12.1	What monitoring is required to be done daily?
12.2	What's the difference between nonviable and viable monitoring?
12.3	What's the difference between certification and monitoring?
12.4	What monitoring is the certifier required to do?
12.5	Our certifier also does the viable testing. Is this OK?
12.6	What should the temperature of the sterile compounding areas be?
12.7	What do I need to do if it's too cold in the sterile compounding area?
12.8	What do I need to do if it's too warm in the sterile compounding area?
12.9	Do I need to monitor the temperature of storage areas outside the intravenous (IV) room?
12.10	What should the humidity be in the sterile compounding area?
12.11	What should I do if the humidity is too low?
12.12	My facilities department says the humidity has to be at least 20%. They want to add a humidifier. Is that OK?
12.13	What should I do if the humidity is too high?
12.14	Can we use a dehumidifier to correct humidity that is too high?
12.15	What should I do if the pressure in my anteroom or positive pressure buffer room is too positive?
12.16	What should I do if the pressure in my negative pressure buffer room or C-SCA is too negative?
12.17	If temperature, humidity, or pressure is out of range, do I have to report this to someone?
12.18	How often does our automated compounding device (ACD) need to be tested?
12.19	How often does our repeater pump need to be tested?

Chapter 13: Certification of Engineering Controls

13.1	What does *certification* mean? How is it different from the monitoring I have to do every day?
13.2	What qualifications does a certifier need?
13.3	What is CETA?
13.4	What are CETA CAGs?
13.5	What should my certification report include?
13.6	What does *dynamic conditions* mean?
13.7 REVISED	Can I compound while the certifier is working in the room?
13.8	Does the certifier need access to the ceiling above the intravenous (IV) room?
13.9	Is there a way to test the ceiling HEPA filters without crawling in the ceiling?
13.10	My hood failed certification. Can I use it?
13.11	My room failed certification. Can I use it?
13.12	We use an ACD. Should we take it out of the hood when the certifier tests the hood?
13.13	We use a repeater pump. Should we take it out of the hood when the certifier tests the hood?
13.14	We use an IV software system that has equipment in the hood. Should we take it out of the hood when the certifier tests the hood?
13.15	Should the certifier do our environmental monitoring?
13.16	If the power goes off in our hood or room, does it need to be recertified before we can use it again?
13.17 REVISED	Our certifier says our chemo room is "too negative." Is this correct?
13.18	Do we have to get our hoods and rooms certified before we use them?

LIST OF QUESTIONS (continued)

LIST OF QUESTIONS (continued)

Chapter 15: Beyond-Use Dates

LIST OF QUESTIONS (continued)

LIST OF QUESTIONS (continued)

LIST OF QUESTIONS (continued)

LIST OF QUESTIONS (continued)

Chapter 18: Environmental Monitoring

LIST OF QUESTIONS (continued)

USP <797> AVAILABILITY

1

1.1 Where can I find the full text of <797>?

United States Pharmacopeial Convention (USP) publishes the *USP Compounding Compendium*.[1] It contains all the major compounding chapters:

- *USP General Chapter <795> Pharmaceutical Compounding—Nonsterile Preparations*[2]
- *USP General Chapter <797> Pharmaceutical Compounding—Sterile Preparations*[3]
- *USP General Chapter <800> Hazardous Drugs—Handling in Healthcare Settings*[4]
- *USP General Chapter <825> Radiopharmaceuticals—Preparation, Compounding, Dispensing, and Repackaging*[5] as well as all the other chapters that are referenced in those core compounding chapters.

Additionally, the General Notices that apply to compounding and compounding monographs are included. The *USP Compounding Compendium* is available through USP at **www.usp.org** as an annual subscription.

1.2 When did <797> become official?

<797> has been an official standard since 2004. It was revised in 2008. Several proposed revisions were published for public comments. The 2023 revision was published on November 1, 2022 with an official date of November 1, 2023.

1.3 Why is there a need for a chapter on sterile compounding? Is this all about the meningitis scare from 2012?

This is a focus on patient safety.[6] It was first published in 2004, so <797> predates the meningitis tragedy of 2012. There were several issues of improper quality (strength as well as microbial contamination) that occurred in 1989 and 1990, prompting both a Food and Drug Administration (FDA) Alert and an ASHP Urgent Attention letter directed to sterile compounders.[7] Those events and others led to the development of <797>.

1.4 Is <797> a guideline? A requirement?

<797> is a minimum standard. Regulators such as federal or state entities can make it a regulation by including it in their documents. Accreditation organizations, such as The Joint Commission, DNV Healthcare, the Accreditation Commission for Health Care, the Center for Improvement in Healthcare Quality, and others, can include it in their own standards.

DOI 10.37573/9781585287260.001

1.5   How can <797> be a minimum standard if my state hasn't incorporated it into regulations?

USP is a standard-setting organization. Even if your state has not codified it into regulation, it is still a federal standard and can be used to inspect or survey your pharmacy.

GENERAL PRINCIPLES OF USP <797> 2

2.1 Is USP <797> a new chapter?

<797> was first published in 2004. It was revised in 2008 and 2023.

2.2 What is the status of the proposed revisions published between 2008 and 2021?

Those were proposed revisions that were published for public comment. New and revised USP chapters are always published for comments which are evaluated and included where appropriate, in the final revision.

2.3 When must I comply with <797>?

<797> is an existing USP General Chapter, so compliance has been required since 2004. Federal and state regulators and accreditation organizations may incorporate USP standards in their own regulations and standards. Check with the organizations with jurisdiction over your site to be sure you comply with their requirements.

2.4 What is the distinction between the terms *must* and *should* in the text of <797>?

USP uses *shall* or *must* for a requirement and *should* for a recommendation. However, some states may expect you to comply with recommendations as well as USP requirements. Consult your state regulations, which may be more stringent than the USP standard.

2.5 If I'm just repackaging sterile products into unit doses, do I need to comply with <797>?

Yes. Repackaging of sterile components is within the scope of <797>. See the FDA document on repackaging.[8]

2.6 Are hazardous drugs addressed in <797>?

Compounding sterile hazardous drugs must comply with both <797> and *USP General Chapter <800> Hazardous Drugs—Handling in Healthcare Settings.*[4] Also see *The Chapter <800> Answer Book*[9] for information on compounding sterile hazardous drugs.

DOI 10.37573/9781585287260.002

2.7   Are radiopharmaceuticals addressed in <797>?

There was a section on radiopharmaceuticals in the 2008 version of <797>, but the information in *USP General Chapter <825> Radiopharmaceuticals—Preparation, Compounding, Dispensing, and Repackaging*[5] supersedes this information.

2.8   Are allergens addressed in <797>?

Yes. Compounding allergenic extracts are within the scope of <797> and addressed in a section of the standard.

CONTENTS OF SECTIONS OF USP <797>

3

USP General Chapter <797> Pharmaceutical Compounding—Sterile Preparations is divided into sections. The key elements in each section are listed below.

Introduction and Scope
- Specific practices
  - Allergenic extracts
  - Biological materials
  - Hazardous drugs
  - Repackaging
  - Radiopharmaceuticals
- Administration
- Immediate use CSPs
- Preparation per approved labeling
- CSP categories

Personnel Training and Evaluation
- Core skills
- Garbing
- Hand hygiene
- Aseptic manipulation competency
  - Media Fill
  - Gloved fingertip and thumb test
  - Surface sampling

Personal Hygiene and Garbing
- Preparation
- Hand hygiene
- Garbing

Facilities and Engineering Controls
- Air quality standards
- Types and design of SECs

DOI 10.37573/9781585287260.003

- ▶ Types and placement of PECs
- ▶ Requirements when using nonsterile starting ingredients
- ▶ Water sources
- ▶ Movement of materials

Certification and Recertification

Microbiological Air and Surface Monitoring

- ▶ Air sampling procedures and action levels
- ▶ Surface sample procedures and action levels

Cleaning, Disinfecting, Applying Sporicidal Disinfectants, and Sterile 70% IPA

- ▶ Agents used
- ▶ Supplies
- ▶ Procedures

Introducing Items into the SEC and PEC

- ▶ Material transfer
- ▶ Use of sIPA on critical sites

Equipment, Supplies, and Components

- ▶ Selection
- ▶ Receipt
- ▶ Evaluation
- ▶ Handling and storage

Sterilization and Depyrogenation

- ▶ Depyrogenation
- ▶ Filters
- ▶ Steam heat
- ▶ Dry heat

Master Formulation and Compounding Records

Release Inspections and Testing

- ▶ Visual inspections
- ▶ Sterility testing
- ▶ Bacterial Endotoxins testing

Labeling

Establishing Beyond-Use Dates

- ▶ Terminology
- ▶ Establishing BUDs

- ▶ Additional requirements for Category 3 CSPs
- ▶ Multiple-dose CSPs

Use of Conventionally Manufactured Products as Components
- ▶ Single-dose containers
- ▶ Multiple-dose containers
- ▶ Pharmacy bulk packages

Use of CSPs as Components
- ▶ Multiple-dose CSPs
- ▶ Single-dose CSPs
- ▶ Stock solutions

Standard Operating Procedures

Quality Assurance and Quality Control
- ▶ Recall of dispensed CSPs
- ▶ Complaints
- ▶ Adverse event reporting

CSP Handling, Storage, Packaging, Shipping, and Transport

Documentation
- ▶ Required documentation
- ▶ Retrievable records

Compounding Allergenic Extracts

Glossary

LIST OF BOXES AND TABLES

Boxes

Section in USP <797>	Number	Title
2.2	1	Gloved Fingertip and Thumb Sampling Procedures
2.3	2	Media-Fill Testing Procedures
3.2	3	Hand Washing Procedures
3.2	4	Hand Sanitizing Procedures
6.2.2	5	Active Air Sampling Procedures for Viable Airborne Monitoring
6.3.2	6	Surface Sampling Procedures
7.2	7	Procedures for Cleaning and Disinfecting the PEC
7.2	8	Procedures for Applying a Sporicidal Disinfectant in the PEC
11.1	9	Master Formulation Records
11.2	10	Compounding Records

Tables

Section in USP <797>	Number	Title
2.3	1	Action Levels for Gloved Fingertip and Thumb Sampling
2.3	2	Initial Training and Competency
2.3	3	Ongoing Training and Competency
4.1.1	4	ISO Classification of Particulate Matter in Room Air
4.2.3	5	Summary of Minimum Requirements for Placement of PECs for Compounding Non-HD CSPs
4.2.4	6	Summary of ACPH Requirements for Non-HD Sterile Compounding Areas
6.2.3	7	Action Levels for Viable Airborne Particle Air Sampling
6.3.3	8	Action Levels for Surface Sampling
7	9	Purpose of Cleaning, Disinfecting, and Sporicidal Disinfectants
7	10	Minimum Frequency for Cleaning and Disinfecting Surfaces and Applying Sporicidal Disinfectants in Classified Areas and the SCA
14.1	11	Summary of Terms
14.3	12	BUD Limits for Category 1 CSPs
14.3	13	BUD Limits for Category 2 CSPs
14.4.4	14	BUD Limits for Category 3 CSPs

SCOPE OF USP <797>

4

4.1   Who has to comply with <797>?

All healthcare personnel who compound sterile preparations must comply with the standards in USP <797>.

4.2   I've heard <797> referred to as a guideline and a standard. Which is correct? What's the difference?

<797> is a federal standard. It's not a guideline; you cannot select certain aspects to consider. You need to follow the entire standard to be compliant.

4.3   Is <797> a regulation?

It is a federal standard. States and other regulatory agencies, accreditation organizations, and health-system policies may include <797> requirements.

4.4   Does <797> apply to animals?

Yes. It applies to sterile compounding for humans and animals.

4.5   Can I select certain sections of <797> to be compliant with?

No. You need to comply with the entire standard.

4.6   Is <797> in effect now?

Yes. It has been since 2004 and was revised in 2008 and 2023.

4.7   What are examples of preparations that must comply—and those that do not comply—with <797>?

Sterile preparations include infusions, injections, aqueous preparations for pulmonary inhalations, irrigations for internal body categories, ophthalmics (including drops), implants, baths and soaks for live organs and tissues. Prepackaging of sterile products and preparations also must comply with <797>. Compounding nasal dosage forms for local application or irrigations for the mouth, rectal cavity, or sinus cavity are not required to be sterile so must comply with <795>.[2]

4.8   Does <797> apply to all compounds?

It applies to all sterile compounds. Nonsterile compounds must comply with <795>.[2] Compounding with hazardous drugs —either nonsterile or sterile—must also comply with <800>.[4]

DOI 10.37573/9781585287260.004

4.9   Does <797> apply to investigational agents?

Yes, if the investigational agent is a sterile compounded preparation. There is also a USP chapter that deals specifically with phase 1 studies: *USP General Chapter <1168> Compounding for Phase 1 Investigational Studies.*[10]

4.10   I work in a hospital pharmacy. Do I need to comply with <795> or <797>?

It depends on the type of preparation. For nonsterile preparations, use <795>. For sterile preparations, use <797>. For hazardous drug (HD) compounding, you also need to comply with <800>. Your nuclear medicine department needs to comply with USP <825>.[5]

4.11   Does <800> replace <797>?

No. <800> provides the information on handling HDs. It must be used in conjunction with <797> for sterile compounding.

4.12   Do community or mail-order pharmacies have to comply with <797>? How about a private physician's office?

All healthcare sites where sterile compounding occurs must comply with <797>. This includes pharmacies of any type, physician offices and clinics, veterinarian offices, and any other healthcare setting where sterile preparations are compounded.

4.13   Do pharmaceutical manufacturers have to comply with <797>?

The scope of <797> is compounding. Manufacturers are under different—and more stringent—requirements to manufacture pharmaceutical products.

4.14   Does a nursing home have to comply with <797>?

The pharmacy provider should be preparing the compounded sterile preparations (CSPs) for the long-term care (LTC) facility. Generally, the activities at an LTC involve preparing sterile products following a manufacturer's approved labeling. That is out of scope of <797> as long as the preparation is for a single patient and will not be stored. However, if sterile compounding is occurring at an LTC facility, those healthcare professionals need to comply with <797>.

4.15   What types of activities aren't considered compounding?

Compounding does not include mixing, reconstituting, or similar acts that are performed in accordance with the directions contained in approved labeling provided by the product's manufacturer and other manufacturer directions consistent with that labeling. This is limited to only nonhazardous drugs and as a single dose for a single patient. The labeling must include the directions for mixing, specific diluent to use (if applicable), the container and closure to use, and the storage time. If that information isn't provided by the manufacturer, the activity is compounding and must comply with <797>.

4.16 How is administering medications distinguished from compounding?

If a dose is prepared for administration (such as by using the manufacturer's instructions) and administered within 4 hours of preparation, it likely meets the definition of Immediate Use. Note that NIOSH Table 1 antineoplastics and other hazardous drugs not entity exempt cannot be prepared as immediate use. (See <800> for additional information about hazardous drugs.[4]) An example of Immediate Use might be an ICU nurse preparing a sodium bicarbonate drip for a stat dose. Of course, they still need to be mixed using aseptic technique by personnel with demonstrated competency to mix immediate use preparations.

4.17 What is the time limit for Immediate Use?

The administration of immediate-use preparations must start within 4 hours of the start of mixing. They do not need to be fully administered within 4 hours; the infusion time limit needs to be set by organizational policy. This is a change from the 2008 version of <797>, which limited immediate use to 1 hour. Since health systems were able to comply with the 1 hour limit, there is no need to change your policy to 4 hours if 1 hour was sufficient. The 4 hour allowance may be applicable in select non-acute areas without pharmacy presence.

4.18 Does <797> include prepackaging from a vial to a unit-dose syringe?

Yes. That meets the definition of compounding in <797>.

4.19 <795> says repackaging is out of scope. Why is it included in <797>?

<797> deals with stability (drug, diluent, container, closure) as well as sterility. Repackaging of a sterile product or preparation from one container to another needs to include the assessment of the change of the container (e.g., vial to syringe) and closure (e.g., manufacturer's vial closure to syringe cap).

4.20 Is it OK to compound a preparation that can be mixed cheaper than the commercial product?

No, if only for the cost issue. See the FDA guidance document *Compounded Drug Products That Are Essentially Copies of Commercially Available Drug Products* under Section 503A of the Federal Food, Drug, and Cosmetic Act.[11]

4.21 Who will enforce <797> for compliance outside of pharmacy settings?

A federal agency can. States determine how they will enforce any standards. Most states have had regulations related to nonsterile compounding for decades and have recently added regulations related to sterile compounding. Accreditation organizations have incorporated <797> in their standards.

HUMAN RESOURCES 5

5.1 DESIGNATED PERSON

5.1-1 Is a compounding supervisor required?

Each compounding site must have one or more individuals identified as the designated person to oversee the responsibilities of compounding sterile preparations. These individuals are responsible for developing and implementing policies and procedures; establishing a training program; overseeing compliance with <797> and any other applicable laws, regulations, and standards; ensuring competency of personnel; selecting components; and ensuring environmental control of the facilities used for storing and compounding CSPs.

5.1-2 Can the designated person be a committee instead of an individual?

There should be at least one person identified as the designated person. That person can lead a committee if that approach is chosen by the entity or could oversee other designated persons.

5.1-3 Does the designated person need to be a pharmacist?

No. It can be anyone qualified to perform the required functions. Healthcare systems will most likely have a pharmacist in this position, but some organizations may assign a pharmacy technician to that function if permitted by state regulations. Some entities (e.g., physician offices, veterinary clinics) may not have a pharmacist available for this function, so will need to assign a qualified person to oversee the compounding functions.

5.1-4 Does the designated person need to be a manager?

No. It is up to the entity to assign the specific person to oversee this.

5.1-5 Is the designated person responsible for compliance with <797>?

Yes. It is a key function of the designated person.

5.1-6 Does oversight of sterile compounding have to be the designated person's sole job responsibility?

No. It is up to the organization to assign job functions.

DOI 10.37573/9781585287260.005

5.1-7   Can the designated person be responsible for more than one site?

Yes. It is up to the entity to assign the responsibility. One person can have responsibility for multiple sites. In multihospital health systems, it is likely that one person would be responsible for oversight of multiple hospitals and other sites that compound.

5.1-8   Where can the designated person obtain the necessary training for this job?

That is up to the entity to define. Training needs to include both didactic and hands-on experience. ASHP offers a certificate program on sterile compounding.[12]

5.1-9   How much training does the designated person need to have?

<797> does not specify the number of hours. Some state regulations require a specific number for relicensure of pharmacists and/or other compounders. The designated person must have a thorough understanding of the standards to be able to develop, implement, and oversee policies, procedures, and practices including personnel training, evaluation, and monitoring as well as facility compliance with <797> and other laws and regulations.

5.1-10   What types of activities is the designated person typically responsible for?

Items include the following:

▶ Compliance with <797>, applicable federal and state laws and regulations, and accreditation standards
▶ Oversight of personnel training, competency documentation, and monitoring
▶ Oversight of facility use and monitoring
▶ Establish standard operating procedures (SOPs)
▶ Develop master formulation records
▶ Monitor beyond-use dates

The designated person needs to monitor and revise the training program to meet changes in services provided and to meet updates in regulations and accreditation standards. In addition to the changes from the 2008 to 2023 version of <797>[13], practices will continue to evolve and need to be addressed.

5.1-11   Does the designated person need to be board-certified?

It is up to the entity to define the requirements. The Board of Pharmacy Specialties (BPS) Certified Sterile Compounding Pharmacist (BCSCP) is a criterion that could be applied.[14] If the designated person is a pharmacy technician, the Pharmacy Technician Certification Board (PTCB) additional distinction of Certified Compounded Sterile Preparation Technician™ (CSPT™) is available and could be included as a criterion.[15] Other certificate programs such as ASHP's Sterile Products Preparation Certificate Program[12] could also be used as a criterion.

5.2 RESPONSIBILITIES OF COMPOUNDING PERSONNEL

5.2-1 What training is required for compounding CSPs?

Education and training concerning sterile compounding need to supplement general education, training, and documentation of competency for handling any drug. *Competence Assessment Tools for Health-System Pharmacies*[16] and ASHP's *Pharmacy Competency Assessment Center*[17] provide checklists and competence documents, including one for compounding sterile preparations. All personnel compounding CSPs need to complete training such as organizational policies and procedures, use of garb, use of equipment, selection of components, and spill management.

Personnel must document initial competency prior to independently compounding CSPs for patients. In order to maintain competence, compounding personnel must requalify by successfully completing garbing and gloved fingertip testing, media fill, post media fill gloved fingertip testing, and surface sampling. Those who mix Category 1 and 2 CSPs must requalify every 6 months and those who mix Category 3 CSPs must requalify every 3 months. Personnel who oversee compounding but do not compound must requalify every 12 months. Other competencies must be documented at least every 12 months.

Other personnel who do not compound (such as those who only restock the sterile compounding area, those who only clean the floors, those who only mix immediate use, etc.) must have competency defined by organizational policy.

5.2-2 What are the key competencies that compounders must demonstrate?

Core competencies include hand hygiene, garbing, knowledge of compounding technique, proper movement of materials, cleaning and disinfection, calculations, measuring and mixing, aseptic technique, achieving and maintaining sterility and apyrogenicity, proper use of equipment, and documentation.[3]

5.3 DOCUMENTING COMPETENCE

5.3-1 What competence information has to be documented?

Competence documents must show that the person can perform functions of the position and that they will comply with your organizational policies and procedures. *Competence Assessment Tools for Health-System Pharmacies*[16] and ASHP's *Pharmacy Competency Assessment Center*[17] provide compounding-related assessments and forms. Assessment of compounding competency requires observation by skilled personnel to ensure proper techniques are followed; be sure to document this observational review and approval. Regulatory inspectors and accreditation organization surveyors often expect tests to have a designated passing score defined in policy.

5.3-2 How often should training occur?

Initial training needs to be completed prior to independently compounding CSPs for patients. Ongoing education and training need to occur whenever new procedures or new equipment is used. Visual observation of hand hygiene and garbing (including successful completion of post-garbing gloved fingertip tests) and successful completion of aseptic processing competencies (including media fill, post media fill gloved fingertip test, and surface sample) must occur at least every 6 months for those mixing Category 1 and 2 CSPs and at least every 3 months for those mixing Category 3 CSPs. Designated persons who oversee compounding but do not compound must complete the tests at least every 12 months. Documentation of ongoing competence for other core competencies needs to occur at least every 12 months.

5.3-3 Is there a set number of training hours required?

There is no such requirement in <797>, although some states have a minimum number of training hours in their regulations.

5.3-4 Do pharmacists who only check—but don't compound—CSPs have to document competency?

It depends. If the pharmacists are in the sterile compounding area observing personnel who compound and may at any point participate in the compounding process, they need to have the same competencies completed as those who routinely compound. However, pharmacists who may perform in-process checks (such as entering orders, viewing in-process photos or videos of steps in the compounding process, or other functions without entering the compounding area) may have competencies defined by organizational policy.

5.3-5 I am at a small hospital and the only pharmacist. How can I document my competency?

You could attend an external training program or have a competent trainer provide education at your site.

5.4 HAZARD COMMUNICATION PLAN

All entities must have a hazard communication plan. This is a requirement of the Occupational Safety and Health Administration (OSHA).

5.4-1 What is a hazard communication plan?

OSHA requires all workplaces where employees are exposed to hazardous chemicals to have a written plan describing how the standard will be implemented in that facility.[18]

5.4.2 Is a hazardous chemical the same thing as a hazardous drug?

Not necessarily. The hazardous drugs (HDs) defined in <800> are those on the National Institute for Occupational Safety and Health (NIOSH) list of HDs.[19] OSHA's hazardous chemical standard includes much more than the NIOSH list because it deals with all types of hazardous chemicals, not just those that are hazardous to healthcare personnel. Review the safety data sheets (SDSs) for chemicals used for compounding and cleaning.

5.4-3 Where can I find safety data sheets?

OSHA requires that chemical manufacturers, distributors, or importers of the hazardous material provide detailed information on the product. SDSs—formerly called material safety data sheets (MSDSs)—provide a structured document that includes the required information you need. You may need to request an SDS from the supplier.

5.4-4 Do all drugs require an SDS?

The raw chemical may require an SDS but some dosage forms are exempt from the requirement.

SDSs are required for the following:

▶ Drugs deemed hazardous by the manufacturer
▶ Solid medications that contain hazardous substances that are intended to be dissolved or crushed before administration

SDSs are not required for the following:

▶ Medications that don't contain hazardous substances
▶ Medications that are in solid, final form for direct administration to the patient
▶ Drugs packaged by the manufacturer for sale to consumers (like over-the-counter medications)

See the OSHA Hazard Communication Standard for further information.[18]

5.4-5 Whose responsibility is it to develop a hazard communication plan?

In a health system, this likely is a function of the Safety Department or other similar department. For small employers that need a summary document, see OSHA's Hazard Communication: *Small Entity Compliance Guide for Employers That Use Hazardous Chemicals.*[20]

POLICIES AND PROCEDURES

6

6.1 What type of policies should I have?

See **Exhibit 6-1.** Your state, accreditation organization, or other agency may require additional policies.

6.2 Are SOPs and policies the same thing?

Policies define the outcome. Procedures explain how things will be done. SOPs is an acronym for standard operating procedures.

6.3 Do the policies have to be written?

Yes. The format is up to you; they can be hard copy or electronic. The key requirement is that they are retrievable.

6.4 Who, and at what frequency, needs to review policies?

Policies need to be reviewed as new sterile products are used, new compounds are made, new equipment is used, or other situations that warrant a review. Minimally, the designated person needs to review policies every 12 months.

6.5 How long do I have to keep old policies?

At least 3 years or longer if required by your jurisdiction, inspecting agency, accreditation organization, or health-system policy.

DOI 10.37573/9781585287260.006

EXHIBIT 6-1. Policies Required and Recommended in USP <797>

Note: If hazardous drugs are compounded, additional policies and procedures are required. See <800>[4] and *The Chapter <800> Answer Book.*[9]

▸ General

  ▲ Standard operating procedures (SOPs) must be written and available to all compounding personnel

  ▲ SOPs must include the types of CSPs prepared (i.e., Category 1, Category 2, Category 3)

  ▲ When compounding activities require the manipulation of a patient's blood-derived or other biological material (e.g., autologous serum), the manipulations must be clearly separated from other compounding activities and equipment used in CSP preparation activities, and they must be controlled by specific standard operating procedures (SOPs) to avoid any cross-contamination. Handling of blood components and other biological materials must additionally comply with laws and regulations of the applicable regulatory jurisdiction

  ▲ A designated person(s) must ensure that SOPs are appropriate and are implemented, which includes ensuring that personnel demonstrate competency in performing every procedure that relates to their job function.

  ▲ A designated person(s) must follow up to ensure that corrective actions are taken if problems, deviations, failures, or errors are identified. The corrective action must be documented.

  ▲ The designated person(s) is responsible for addressing other areas of risk in the facility's SOPs.

  ▲ All personnel who perform or oversee compounding or support activities must be trained in the SOPs, including

    » Recognize potential problems, deviations, failures, or errors associated with preparing a CSP (e.g., those related to equipment, facilities, materials, personnel, the compounding process, or testing) that could potentially result in contamination or other adverse impact on CSP quality

    » Report any problems, deviations, failures or errors to the designated person(s) SOPs must be reviewed initially and at least every 12 months by the designated person(s) to ensure that they reflect current practices, and the review must be documented.

  ▲ Any changes or alterations to an SOP must be made only by a designated person(s) and must be documented.

  ▲ Revisions to SOPs must be communicated to all personnel involved in these processes and procedures, and personnel should document acknowledgment of the communication.

▸ Documentation

  ▲ All facilities where CSPs are prepared must have and maintain written or electronic documentation to demonstrate compliance with the requirements in this chapter. This documentation must include, but is not limited to, the following:

    » Personnel training, competency assessments, and qualification records including corrective actions for any failures

EXHIBIT 6-1. (cont'd)

» Certification reports, including corrective actions for any failures

» Environmental air and surface monitoring procedures and results

» Equipment records (e.g., calibration, verification, and maintenance reports)

» Receipt of components

» SOPs

» Master Formulation Records (MFRs) (if required)

» Compounding Records (CRs) (if required)

» All required CRs for a particular CSP (e.g., MFR, CR, and release inspection and testing results) must be readily retrievable for at least 2 years after preparation or as required by laws and regulations of the applicable regulatory jurisdiction or accrediting organization(s), whichever is longer

» Release inspection and testing records

» Information related to complaints and adverse events including corrective actions taken

» Results of investigations and corrective actions

» Documentation must comply with all laws and regulations of the applicable regulatory jurisdiction

▲ Records must be legible and stored in a manner that prevents their deterioration and/or loss.

▶ Personnel Training

▲ All training must be documented

▲ Personnel compounding only immediate-use CSPs must complete training as required by the facility's SOPs. Immediate use SOPs include aseptic techniques, processes, and procedures to be followed, minimize the potential for contact with nonsterile surfaces, introduction of particulate matter or biological fluids, and mix-ups with other conventionally manufactured products or CSPs.

▲ Personnel who only perform restocking or cleaning and disinfecting duties outside of the PEC must complete ongoing training as required by the facility's SOPs

▲ Processes and techniques for handling, storing, packaging, and transporting CSPs must be outlined in the facility's SOPs. Personnel who will be handling, storing, packaging, and transporting CSPs within the facility must be trained in accordance with the relevant SOPs, and the training must be documented.

▲ A written training program must describe the required training, the frequency of training, and the process for evaluating the performance of individuals who compound, have direct oversight of compounding personnel, perform in-process checks, final verification, and dispensing of CSPs. This program must equip personnel with the appropriate knowledge and train them in the required skills necessary to perform their assigned tasks, and SOPs specify the training required for such task.

▲ Initial training for compounders, designated persons, and personnel with direct oversight of compounding must include

» Training and competency in maintaining the quality of the sterile compounding environment

EXHIBIT 6-1. (cont'd)

- » Training and competency in sterile compounding principles and practices
- » Garbing competency including gloved fingertip test (GFT)
- » Media fill with post GFT and surface sampling
- ▲ Initial training must be defined by facility personnel for
  - » Personnel who do not compound but who restock or clean and disinfect the sterile compounding areas
  - » Personnel who perform in-process checks or final verification of CSPs
  - » Personnel who only compound immediate use CSPs
  - » Others, such as maintenance personnel, certifiers, contractors, inspectors, surveyors, etc.
- ▲ Ongoing training and competency for compounders must include
  - » At least every 12 months
    - ▼ Training and competency in sterile compounding principles and practices
  - » At least every 6 months for those who compound Category 1 and/or Category 2 CSPs
    - ▼ Garbing competency (including GFT)
    - ▼ Media fill with post GFT and surface sampling
  - » At least every 3 months for those who compound Category 3 CSPs
    - ▼ Garbing competency (including GFT)
    - ▼ Media fill with post GFT and surface sampling
- ▲ For those designated persons and personnel with direct oversight of compounding who do not compound, ongoing training and competency must be completed at least every 12 months and must include
  - » Training and competency in sterile compounding principles and practices
  - » Garbing competency (including GFT)
  - » Media fill with post GFT and surface sampling
- ▲ Ongoing training must be defined by facility personnel for
  - » Personnel who do not compound but who restock or clean and disinfect the sterile compounding areas
  - » Personnel who perform in-process checks or final verification of CSPs
  - » Personnel who only compound immediate use CSPs
  - » Others, such as maintenance personnel, certifiers, contractors, inspectors, surveyors, etc.
- ▶ Garbing
  - ▲ The required garb, manner of storage, and order of garbing must be determined by the facility and documented in the facility's SOPs
  - ▲ The facility's SOPs must describe disinfection procedures for reusing goggles, respirators, and other reusable equipment

EXHIBIT 6-1. (cont'd)

- ▶ RABS sleeves and gloves
  - ▲ The RABS sleeves and gloves and the pharmaceutical isolator sleeves and gloves should be changed per the manufacturer's recommendations and as defined in the facility's SOPs.
- ▶ Components
  - ▲ Compounding personnel must follow the facility's SOPs, which must address the selection, receipt, evaluation, handling, storage, and documentation of all CSP components, including all ingredients and container closure
  - ▲ Weighing, measuring, or otherwise manipulating components that could generate airborne chemical particles (e.g., active pharmaceutical ingredients [APIs], added substances, conventionally manufactured products) must be evaluated to determine if these activities must be performed in a PEC or other closed system processing device (e.g., single use containment glove bag) to reduce the potential exposure to personnel or contamination of the facility or CSPs. The process evaluation must be carried out in accordance with the facility's SOPs and the assessment must be documented.
- ▶ Equipment
  - ▲ Compounding personnel must follow established SOPs for the calibration, maintenance, cleaning, and use of the equipment based on the manufacturer's recommendations.
- ▶ Incubation Temperature
  - ▲ The incubator temperature must be monitored during incubation, either manually or by a continuous recording device, and the results must be reviewed and documented as described in the facility's SOPs.
  - ▲ The order of the incubation temperatures for media fill must be described in the facility's SOPs.
- ▶ Master Formulation Records (MFRs)
  - ▲ Any changes or alterations to the MFR must be approved and documented according to the facility's SOPs
- ▶ Terminal Sterilization (if performed)
  - ▲ A description of the terminal sterilization and depyrogenation process, including the temperature, pressure (if applicable), duration, permissible load conditions for each cycle, and the use of biological indicators and endotoxin challenge vials (ECVs) must be included in the facility's SOPs. SOPs must include training and competency of personnel on all sterilization methods and equipment used by the facility. In addition, the SOPs must include a schedule and method for establishing and verifying the effectiveness of the terminal sterilization and depyrogenation methods selected, as well as the methods for maintaining and cleaning the sterilizing and depyrogenation equipment
  - ▲ The effectiveness of the depyrogenation cycle must be re-established if there are changes to the depyrogenation cycle described in SOPs (e.g., changes in load conditions, duration, or temperature). This verification must be documented,
- ▶ Labeling
  - ▲ Labeling procedures must be followed as described in the facility's SOPs to prevent labeling errors and CSP mix-ups.

EXHIBIT 6-1. (cont'd)

▲ The label of the CSP must be verified to ensure that it conforms with the: Prescription or medication order; MFR, if required; and CR

▶ Nonviable Monitoring

  ▲ The temperature and humidity readings must be reviewed as described in the facility's SOPs.

  ▲ All total airborne sampling sites and procedures must be described in the facility's SOPs

  ▲ The results of the temperature readings must be documented in a temperature log per facility SOPs or stored in the continuous temperature recording device and must be retrievable.

  ▲ Temperature monitoring devices must be verified for accuracy at least every 12 months or as required by the manufacturer

▶ Viable Monitoring

  ▲ Sterile compounding facilities must develop and implement written procedures for microbiological air and surface monitoring

  ▲ The microbiological air and surface monitoring program must be clearly described in the facility's SOPs, which must include a diagram of the sampling locations, procedures for collecting samples, frequency of sampling, size of samples (e.g., surface area, volume of air), time of day of sampling in relation to activities in the compounding area, and action levels that will trigger corrective action

  ▲ All sampling sites and procedures must be described in the facility's SOPs

▶ Cleaning

  ▲ All cleaning and disinfecting activities must be performed by trained and appropriately garbed personnel using facility-approved agents and procedures, which must be described in written SOPs.

  ▲ The frequency, method(s), and location(s) of cleaning, disinfecting, and applying sporicidal disinfectants must be established in written SOPs, in accordance with the manufacturer's instructions and must be followed by all cleaning personnel. The manufacturer's directions or published data for minimum contact time must be followed for each of the cleaning, disinfecting, and sporicidal disinfectants used.

  ▲ When sterile 70% IPA is used, it must be allowed to dry. All cleaning, disinfecting, and application of sporicidal disinfectants must be documented according to the facility's SOP.

  ▲ Once opened, sterile cleaning and disinfecting agents and supplies (e.g., closed containers of sterile wipers,) and sterile 70% IPA may be reused for a time period specified as by the manufacturer and/or described in the facility written SOP.

▶ Release testing

  ▲ All release testing procedures (e.g., visual inspections and testing) must be included in the facility's documentation for MFRs and CRs

  ▲ Visual inspection defects which indicate sterility or stability problems must be investigated to determine the cause according to the facility's SOPs

EXHIBIT 6-1. (cont'd)

▶ Quality Assurance and Quality Control Program

▲ A facility's QA and QC programs must be formally established and documented in the facility's SOPs that ensure that all aspects of the preparation of CSPs are conducted in accordance with the requirements in this chapter <797>, and laws and regulations of the applicable regulatory jurisdiction.

▲ The facility's SOPs must describe the roles, duties, and training of the personnel responsible for each aspect of the QA program. Designated person(s) responsible for the QA program must have the training, experience, responsibility, and authority to perform these duties. The overall QA and QC program must be reviewed at least once every 12 months by the designated person(s). The results of the review must be documented, and appropriate action must be taken if needed

▲ An SOP for recall of out-of-specification dispensed CSPs must contain:

» Procedures to determine the severity of the problem and the urgency for implementation and completion of the recall.

» Procedures to determine the distribution of any affected CSP, including the date and quantity of distribution.

» Procedures to identify patients who have received the CSP.

» Procedures for disposal and documentation of the recalled CSP.

» Procedures to investigate and document the reason for failure.

▲ The sterile compounding facility must document the implementation of the recall procedures. The recall must be reported to appropriate regulatory bodies as required by laws and regulations of the applicable regulatory jurisdiction.

▲ Compounding facilities must develop and implement SOPs for handling complaints.

▲ Adverse events potentially associated with the quality of CSPs must be reported in accordance with the facility's SOPs and all laws and regulations of the applicable regulatory jurisdiction.

GARB AND HAND HYGIENE 7

7.1 GENERAL INFORMATION

7.1-1 What does <797> require for garb?

The components of required garb include gowns or coveralls, gloves, hair covers, masks, and shoe covers. If you are compounding hazardous compounded sterile preparations (CSPs), additional personal protective equipment (PPE) is required. See <800>[4] and *The Chapter <800> Answer Book*[9] for details.

The garbing procedure—the order in which garb is donned—needs to be developed and detailed in your policies and needs to match the facility design (such as placement of the sink) you have.

7.1-2 What is the purpose of garb?

Garb provides protection for the preparation you are compounding.

7.1-3 What is the difference between garb and PPE?

Think of *garb* as protection for the preparation you are compounding and *PPE* as protection for the compounder.

7.1-4 Is different garb required for hazardous and nonhazardous CSPs?

Some of the components are the same, such as hair covers, shoe covers, and masks. Specific types of gloves and gowns must be worn when mixing antineoplastics (and other hazardous drugs if they are not entity-exempt through the organization's Assessment of Risk). See <800>[4] and *The Chapter <800> Answer Book*[9] for details for PPE requirements and recommendations when compounding hazardous drugs. Chemotherapy (commonly known as "chemo") gowns and sterile chemo gloves can be used when compounding nonhazardous CSPs, but they also need to meet the requirements of garb for compounding nonhazardous CSPs.

7.1-5 Is additional garb required for personnel who are compounding from powders?

This needs to be addressed in your policies and procedures. There is additional eye and respiratory risk when working with active pharmaceutical ingredients (APIs) and other raw materials.

DOI 10.37573/9781585287260.007

7.1-6   Do I need to wear garb if the hood I work in is a glove box?

Yes. Garb as described in <797> must be worn when using any type of PEC, including a CAI or CACI.

7.1-7   What does *donning* and *doffing* mean?

Don means to put on PPE; *doff* means to remove it.

7.1-8   Does the pharmacist who is only checking items need to garb?

It depends on the location where checking occurs. Whoever is in the sterile compounding area needs to be appropriately garbed. It doesn't matter if they are compounding, checking, observing, certifying, cleaning, repairing equipment, or any other activity.

7.1-9   Can garb be reused?

Gowns used for nonhazardous compounding—if not torn, soiled, contaminated, or otherwise compromised—can be carefully removed and hung up inside the anteroom or inside or adjacent to the segregated compounding area (SCA) for use for the remainder of the shift for use by the same person. Other disposable garb must not be reused. Reusable garb (such as goggles) must be cleaned and disinfected after use.

7.1-10   The pharmacists and technicians who work in our operating room (OR) satellite wear "OR greens." Is this sufficient garb?

It depends what they are doing. If you are preparing intravenous (IV) mixtures in an SCA, you need the additional garb required. If you are mixing an IV for immediate use, it may be sufficient based on your policies.

7.2 HAND HYGIENE

7.2-1   What does *hand hygiene* mean?

The Centers for Disease Control and Prevention (CDC) defines *hand hygiene* as "cleaning your hands by using either handwashing (washing hands with soap and water), antiseptic hand wash, antiseptic hand rub (i.e., alcohol-based hand sanitizer including foam or gel), or surgical hand antisepsis." Prior to compounding, you need to wash your hands with soap and water. Use of only alcohol hand sanitizers is not enough. See the CDC's Hand Hygiene in Healthcare Settings[21] guidelines for further information.

7.2-2   Can alcohol-based hand rub be used instead of soap and water?

No. It is not a replacement for soap and water. Alcohol-based hand rub is used as part of the hand hygiene and garbing procedure.

7.2-3   How long should our policy say to wash hands?

Prior to compounding, wash your hands and forearms with soap and water for at least 30 seconds.

7.2-4 Are regular paper towels OK to use?

No. Use low-linting disposable towels or wipers.

7.3 GLOVES

7.3-1 When gloves are mentioned in <797>, what kind of gloves does that mean?

Sterile, powder-free gloves. If hazardous CSPs are compounded, gloves that meet ASTM Standard D6978 are required.[22]

7.3-2 Is it OK to wash gloves between compounds?

No. If gloves are soiled or contaminated, they need to be discarded and new gloves donned.

7.3-3 When are sterile gloves required?

Sterile gloves are required when compounding CSPs and when entering the buffer room of a cleanroom suite or inside the perimeter around the PEC in an SCA or C-SCA.

7.3-4 We use glove boxes to put on gloves outside of the glove box. Is this correct?

No. When using compounding isolators, you need to pass the sterile gloves through the antechamber and don them inside the compounding aseptic isolator (CAI) or compounding aseptic containment isolator (CACI) over the gloves on the compounding isolator sleeves.

7.3-5 Are sterile gloves required when working in a compounding isolator?

Yes. A sterile glove needs to be the one that touches the preparation. *You need a minimum of two pairs of gloves:* one on the compounding isolator sleeve(that should be changed at least daily) and another pair for the compounder. Those gloves must be passed through the antechamber and donned inside the CAI. You may also want to use another disposable pair of gloves to use on your hands inside the gloves accessed through the compounding isolator sleeve.

7.3-6 How often do compounding isolator gloves need to be changed?

The gloves connected to the sleeves should be changed per the manufacturer's recommendations, as defined by the facility policy, and if they are torn or punctured or if you know or suspect they have been contaminated. They also need to be changed if compounders use different size gloves as their gloves would not fit over the CAI gloves.

7.3-7 Do chemo gloves have to meet a particular standard?

Yes. Chemotherapy ("chemo") gloves used for handling hazardous drugs (HDs) must meet ASTM Standard D6978, the *Standard Practice for Assessment of Resistance of Medical Gloves to Permeation by Chemotherapy Drugs.*[22] Some gloves are tested only for permeation to general chemicals using ASTM F739-12e1 (*Standard Test Method for Permeation of Liquids and Gases through Protective Clothing Materials under Conditions of Continuous Contact*[23]), which is not sufficient for HD gloves.

7.3-8 How do I know if a glove is chemo-rated?

Documentation that the gloves meet ASTM D6978 needs to be listed on the product labeling. It can generally be found on the box of the gloves.

7.3-9 Is it OK for chemo gloves to be tested per ASTM D6978 and laboratory chemical tested per ASTM F739?

Yes, as long as they document that they meet the ASTM Standard D6978.

7.4 GOWNS

7.4-1 Do gowns have to be sterile?

<797> does not require sterile gowns for compounding Category 1 or 2 CSPs.

For compounding Category 3 CSPs, all outer garb must be sterile and low-lint, including sterile sleeves over the gauntlet sleeves on a CAI or CACI (if used).

7.4-2 What is the difference between gowns we use for non-HDs and those used for chemo?

Gowns used for handling antineoplastic agents must be impervious. Gowns used for non-HDs can be made of other materials, depending on their intended use. Your entity's Assessment of Risk may allow different gowns when handling HDs that are not National Institute for Occupational Safety and Health (NIOSH) Table 1 antineoplastic agents.[19]

7.4-3 Can I hang my gown in the anteroom for use later in the day?

Yes, if it was used for nonhazardous drug preparation and is not soiled or otherwise compromised. If your policy allows, you can reuse the gown within the same shift by the same person as long as it is hung inside the classified area or inside or adjacent to the SCA. Gowns used to mix chemo cannot be reused.

7.4-4 Are washable gowns OK to use?

Yes for Category 1 or 2 CSPs if they are low-linting, have sleeves that fit snugly around the wrist, and are enclosed at the neck. However, consider use of disposable gowns. If you use washable gowns, a clean gown needs to be donned daily and whenever soiled or contaminated. For Category 3 CSPs, <797> allows reusable gowns provided they are laundered and resterilized with a validated cycle.

7.4-5 Do I need to wear a regular gown under my chemo gown?

That is not specified in <797>, but think about your facility design and work practices. If you are in a sterile compounding suite, you need to have a regular gown under your chemo gown because you will be entering the clean side of your anteroom when you exit your negative pressure buffer room. You have to be properly gowned at that point, so you need to have on a gown, gloves, mask, hair cover, and shoe covers.

If your HD facility is a containment segregated compounding area (C-SCA) or an area devoted to nonsterile compounding, you may not need a regular gown because you will be exiting into a general pharmacy area. However, think of your containment practices. Consider using a regular gown even in these situations to further protect your clothing.

7.5 HAIR COVERS

7.5-1 What is the difference between head and beard covers used for chemo and those used for nonhazardous CSPs?

There is no difference. The same products can be used for handling HDs as you use for handling non-HDs.

7.5-2 One of our employees is completely bald. Does he need to wear a hair cover?

Yes. It's to cover the head as well as hair. Humans still shed particles and that's what head and hair covers are intended to mitigate.

7.5-3 If personnel wear a head cover for religious or other reasons, is an additional hair cover necessary?

Yes. The purpose of the hair cover is to protect the preparation from potential microbial contamination. Hair covers come in various formats, including bouffants and hoods. The additional head/hair covers must be placed over the head cover worn for religious or other reasons.

7.5-4 Do earrings have to be removed, or can they just be covered by the hair cover?

They need to be removed. <797> requires removal of piercings that could interfere with the effectiveness of garbing. Earrings could get caught on the hair cover, and they also could be a contamination risk.

7.6 MASKS

7.6-1 Do I have to wear a surgical mask when compounding?

A surgical or procedural mask is required for sterile compounding. However, a mask is *not* respiratory protection; it protects the preparation, not the compounder.

7.6-2 Is a mask the same thing as a respirator?

No. The surgical or procedural mask is worn to protect the preparation you are mixing. It does not protect your respiratory system. A respirator, which also functions as a mask, provides respiratory protection to the compounder.

7.6-3 Is a face shield a mask?

They are not the same. You still need a mask when wearing a face shield, unless you use a combined mask/face shield.

7.7 SLEEVES

7.7-1 Are sleeve covers required?

No, but they can be used if required by your policy.

7.8 SHOE COVERS

7.8-1 What is the difference between shoe covers used for chemo and those used for non-HDs?

There is no difference. The same low-lint products can be used for handling HDs as you use for handling non-HDs. However, you may want to consider using shoe covers that are impervious.

7.8-2 Can I use dedicated cleanroom shoes instead of shoe covers?

Shoe covers are required in cleanroom suites, SCAs, and C-SCAs. Any shoes—including those that may be dedicated to the cleanroom—must be covered with shoe covers.

7.9 EYE PROTECTION

7.9-1 What does *eye protection* mean?

When eye protection is needed, it needs to be provided by using goggles. Goggles fit tightly, covering the eyes, eye sockets, and facial area surrounding the eyes. Goggles can be obtained that fit over eyeglasses.

7.9-2 I wear prescription eyeglasses. Does this qualify as eye protection?

No. Eyeglasses alone do not protect against splashes to the eyes. You need to obtain goggles that fit over your eyeglasses if eye protection is needed.

7.9-3 I wear a face shield to protect my contact lenses from drying out. Is this proper eye protection?

Face shields can be used to supplement other garb as long as it is not prohibited by your policy. Face shields alone do not protect against splashes to the eyes. You have to wear goggles when eye protection is needed.

7.9-4 Do I need eye protection when I'm cleaning up a spill?

Yes. Wear eye protection when cleaning up a spill.

7.10 RESPIRATORY PROTECTION

7.10-1 What does *respiratory protection* mean?

When respiratory protection is needed, a fit-tested NIOSH-certified N95 or more protective respirator is generally adequate to protect against airborne particles. However, N95 respirators don't protect against gases or vapors and provide only limited protection against direct liquid splashes. See the NIOSH page on Respirator Trusted-Source Information[24] for more information.

7.10-2 What does an N95 respirator protect against?

It provides protection against airborne particles. It does not protect against gases or vapors.

7.10-3 Are there respirators that are better protection than N95?

There are other respirators that may meet your needs, which you should determine at your organization. Other types include full face-piece, chemical cartridge-type respirators, elastomeric half-mask respirators with multigas cartridges and P100 filters (or a cartridge targeted to the specific drug), or powered air purifying respirators (PAPRs).

7.10-4 Do surgical masks provide adequate respiratory protection?

Surgical or procedural masks do not provide respiratory protection from drug exposure and must not be used alone when respiratory protection is required.

7.10-5 Because the biological safety cabinet (BSC) and compounding aseptic containment isolator (CACI) provide respiratory protection, do I need to wear a regular mask for any HD compounding?

Yes. You need a surgical or procedural mask when compounding any sterile preparation.

7.10-6 Do I need respiratory protection when I'm cleaning up a spill?

Yes. Respiratory protection is needed when cleaning up a spill. Your policy needs to define the PPE required when cleaning up a spill.

7.11 GARBING PROCEDURES

7.11-1 What garb components are garbed first?

The order of garbing depends on the placement of your sink and your workflow. It needs to be defined to minimize potential contamination. Your policy needs to clearly list the components and order of garbing. Personnel need to be observed initially and at the requalifying intervals (at least every 6 months for those mixing Category 1 or 2 CSPs, at least every 3 months for those mixing Category 3 CSPs, and at least every 12 months for designated persons who do not compound). The review needs to be documented.

7.11-2 We put on hair covers, shoe covers, and masks before entering the clean side of the anteroom. In what order should these be donned?

It doesn't matter (unless required by your state), but the order must be detailed in your policy and followed. The order of garbing depends on the location of your sink and your workflow. Many organizations enter the dirty side of the anteroom, don these three components of garb, then step over into the clean side of the anteroom to wash hands, don gown, use alcohol-based hand rub on hands, and then don sterile gloves. Define the components of garb and order of garbing in your policy and be sure the policy is followed by all who enter the compounding area.

7.11-3 What is the proper order of donning garb for compounding CSPs in a cleanroom suite (positive pressure anteroom with sink on the clean side of the anteroom and positive pressure buffer room)?

Your policies and procedures need to describe the garbing sequence based on your facility design. Gowns, shoe covers, head/hair covers, and face masks need to be low-lint.

One option to don garb for the facility design described in the question:

1. Enter dirty side of anteroom.
2. Don mask, hair cover, and shoe covers.
3. Step over into clean side of anteroom.
4. Wash hands.
5. Don gown.
6. Apply alcohol-based hand rub.
7. Don sterile gloves.

7.11-4 What is the proper order of donning garb for compounding CSPs in an SCA with a sink inside the room but outside the perimeter around the PEC?

Your policies and procedures need to describe the garbing sequence based on your facility design. Gowns, shoe covers, head/hair covers, and face masks need to be low-lint.

One option to don garb for the facility design described in the question:

1. Enter SCA, remaining outside the perimeter around the PEC.
2. Don mask, hair cover, and shoe covers.
3. Wash hands.
4. Don gown.
5. Step over the perimeter line.
6. Apply alcohol-based hand rub.
7. Don sterile gloves.

7.11-5 My facility design is different from the two examples above. Do I need to use only the order listed?

No. Your garbing procedure needs to match the design of your facility, particularly the location of your sink. Don garb in an order that reduces the risk of contamination.

7.11-6 Is additional garb required for personnel who are compounding from powders?

This should be considered in your policies and practices. There is additional eye and respiratory risk when working with APIs and other raw materials.

IMMEDIATE USE AND PREPARATION FOR ADMINISTRATION

8

8.1 What is considered *immediate use?*

In situations when compounding cannot occur in a <797>-compliant area, immediate-use preparations may be mixed. These immediate-use preparations do not necessarily need to comply with the facility or monitoring requirements detailed in <797>. Of course, for patient safety and consistency, these preparations should be compounded in compliant areas, but <797> allows for this for patient care needs. Acute care situations present where doses are needed stat for critical patients or a CSP is needed during a procedure that was unanticipated.

NIOSH Table 1 antineoplastic drugs[19] cannot be mixed as immediate-use preparations.

All of the following conditions must be met for a CSP to be considered immediate use:

▶ Written procedures are in place.

▶ The personnel mixing immediate-use preparations are aware of the organization's policy limitations and have documented competence to comply with the policies.

▶ Aseptic procedures are followed.

▶ Compatibility of the components are known.

▶ Only manufacturer's original containers are used as part of the preparation.

▶ The mixture contains no more than three different sterile products.

▶ Single-dose containers must be used for only one patient and cannot be saved for future use.

▶ The CSP is labeled, including the ingredients, preparer, and beyond-use time (which cannot exceed 4 hours from the start of preparation).

8.2 What is considered *administration?*

<797> is about compounding, so administration of medications is not in scope of the chapter.

The information in the Centers for Disease Control and Prevention (CDC) Safe Injection Practices document[25] and related references should be used to establish the organization's policies concerning administration of sterile products and preparations.

8.3 What is considered *preparation for administration?*

Medications such as injections often contain instructions for preparation in FDA-approved labeling. This applies only to those medications that will be prepared for a single dose for a single patient that will be used right away and the specific instructions in

DOI 10.37573/9781585287260.008

the labeling are used. To meet this provision, the labeling must include the amount of the specific diluent to use, the strength of the final concentration, the type of container to use (such as a syringe or an IV bag), and the storage time allowed. If these details are not available, the full information in <797> must be followed.

8.4   Can nurses mix compounded sterile preparations (CSPs) for immediate use?

Yes. Any qualified health professional can mix an immediate-use preparation as long as it is within their scope of practice, your policy allows it, and they have documented competency.

8.5   Can staff other than nurses mix CSPs for immediate use?

Yes. Any qualified health professional can mix an immediate-use preparation as long as it is within their scope of practice, your policy allows it, and they have documented competency.

8.6   Can pharmacy personnel mix CSPs for immediate use?

Yes. Any qualified health professional can mix an immediate-use preparation as long as your policy allows, and they have documented competency.

8.7   Is reconstitution of an antibiotic vial considered immediate use or preparation for administration?

It depends on what is done with the reconstituted drug. If given immediately as an injection, it is preparation for administration. If mixed into an IV solution, using specific instructions in the product labeling include the specific diluent, IV solution base, and final concentration, it is *immediate use.* From a practical perspective in this situation, it depends on the limitations of your organizational policy.

8.8   If a nurse reconstitutes an antibiotic and places it in a piggyback, is this immediate use?

Is this an urgent situation? It should be done by pharmacy in a <797>-compliant area if possible. If it is a stat (or perhaps the first dose of an antibiotic at night when pharmacy is closed), it can be done if allowed by your policy, the nurse has documented competence for this, and it doesn't exceed the limitations of immediate use. Immediate use preparations are limited to no more than three different sterile products. Chemo and other hazardous drugs not exempt in your Assessment of Risk cannot be mixed as immediate use preparations.

8.9   What's the difference between using three sterile containers and using three different sterile products?

Here's an example: a nurse in the intensive care unit (ICU) needs to mix three vials of sodium bicarbonate into a liter bag of an IV solution for a stat dose. This is four containers and three entries into any one container, which exceeded the allowable limits of immediate use in the 2008 version of <797>. This mixture is permitted under the 2023 revision of <797> because it involves two different sterile products (the IV bag and the drug).

8.10 How long after someone mixes an immediate-use IV does it have to be used?

Administration of the CSP must be started within 4 hours of mixing. Note that administration must begin within 4 hours; the IV does not have to be fully administered within 4 hours. Your organizational policy needs to define the allowances for infusion ("hang") time. There is no requirement to change your policy from 1 hour to 4 hours. Most acute care organizations complied with the 1 hour limit so do not need to change their policy.

8.11 Does an immediate-use IV need to be hung within 1 or 4 hours of preparation?

An immediate use preparation needs to be started as soon as possible after mixing. The 2023 revision of <797> allows that to occur within 4 hours. The previous version of <797> limited this to 1 hour.

8.12 I thought immediate use meant to use it right away. Do we have to wait 4 hours after mixing to hang the IV?

It does mean to use it right away. The immediate-use provision is included in <797> to allow for the stat doses that are required for patient care. Because <797> applies to all sites where CSPs are made, there may be some procedural or nonacute sites where some additional time is necessary.

8.13 Can a Banana Bag be mixed under the immediate-use definition?

It depends on the content. Generally, such a mixture includes a base solution, folic acid, thiamine, and multiple vitamins. If that is the case, that is four components so outside of the definition of immediate use. Many organizations have approached this situation by running the thiamine via a secondary IV for the first bag then mixing subsequent bags in <797>-compliant areas.

8.14 Is it OK to let the night nursing supervisors enter the pharmacy to use the IV hood?

No. Nursing can mix the IVs necessary for immediate use without the need to access the sterile compounding area. If they do use the hood, they need to comply with all the requirements of compounding personnel.

8.15 Our pharmacy is not open 24 hours. The nurses in ICU occasionally need to mix a sodium bicarbonate IV stat. Is this OK using the immediate-use definition?

The organizational policy must allow it; they need to have documented competency, and the CSP is limited to no more than three different sterile products.

8.16   When anesthesia staff prepare syringes for cases, is this the immediate-use provision?

Yes. If syringes are prepared for a case in the OR (so, outside a <797>-compliant area), they meet the immediate-use provision.

8.17   Do nurses and anesthesia personnel need to complete the same competency to mix IVs that pharmacists and pharmacy techs need to do?

If they mix only immediate-use CSPs, they do not need to complete the garbing gloved fingertip test or the aseptic processing tests (media fill, post media fill gloved fingertip test, and surface sample) listed in <797>, but they must have successfully completed the competencies defined by the organization.

8.18   Do personnel who prepare only immediate-use IVs need to complete a media fill and gloved fingertip and thumb test?

If they mix only immediate-use CSPs, they do not need to complete the media fill, gloved fingertip and thumb test, or surface sampling requirements. However, they must have documented competence to mix immediate-use CSPs.

8.19   Our pre-op area spikes a case of liters of Lactated Ringers for the following morning use. Is this OK under the immediate-use provision?

IV bags are single-use containers that do not contain preservatives. Administration is out of scope of <797> but consider the infection control risks. See the Association for Professionals in Infection Control and Epidemiology (APIC) position paper on Safe Infection, Infusion, and Medication Vial Practices in Healthcare[26] for further information.

8.20   One of our physicians is a dermatologist. Her staff prepares buffered lidocaine syringes for the day's use. Is this OK under the immediate-use provision?

See the definition of immediate use to be sure the preparation meets the definition. An entire day's worth would not be acceptable because there is a limit of 4 hours between mixing and administration.

8.21   One of our physician's offices has an allergy clinic. His staff mixes allergen extracts for patient use. Is this OK under the immediate-use provision?

The immediate-use provision doesn't apply in this situation, but there is a section in <797> that deals with requirements for preparation of allergen extracts. (See 11.14.)

PERSONNEL TRAINING AND COMPETENCE DOCUMENTATION

9

9.1 INITIAL TRAINING

9.1-1 What initial training is required to mix compounded sterile preparations (CSPs)?

Personnel must be trained by a qualified person and demonstrate competency. A number of core competencies are required by <797> and you will need to supplement those with your organizational-specific requirements.

9.1-2 What are the core competencies that a compounder must demonstrate?

Include these items in the training:

▸ Hand hygiene
▸ Garbing
▸ Calculations
▸ Measuring and mixing
▸ Moving products and supplies throughout the compounding space
▸ Aseptic technique
▸ Negative pressure technique (if hazardous drugs are compounded)
▸ Use of primary engineering controls
▸ Maintenance of secondary engineering controls
▸ Use of closed system drug-transfer devices (if used)
▸ Use of equipment and supplies
▸ Theoretical principles of air flow
▸ Use of autoclaves (if nonsterile-to-sterile preparations are mixed)
▸ Required documentation
▸ Cleaning and disinfection

9.1-3 Should I hire only personnel with prior IV room experience?

That is up to you but you need to be sure that any personnel who compound are competent to do so. *Competency* is a combination of demonstration of core and other competencies, completion of hand hygiene and garbing competencies (including

DOI 10.37573/9781585287260.009

garbing gloved fingertip test), completion of aseptic processing competencies (media fill, post media fill gloved fingertip test, and surface sample), and knowledge of your organizational policies and procedures.

9.1-4   If people have documented training from other hospitals, do I need to train them?

Some training may be transferable between sites but they must be able to demonstrate successful completion of the same competencies you require for any compounder and demonstrate knowledge of your organizational policies and procedures. You need to be sure that the techniques used are correct.[27]

9.1-5   What resources are available for training materials?

<797> lists the basic requirements. Didactic training[12,17] and a number of resources are available from ASHP. See **Exhibit 9-1**.

EXHIBIT 9-1. Sterile Compounding Resources Available from ASHP

Resource Center

▶   Sterile Compounding Resource Center at **www.ashp.org**

Guidelines

▶   Compounding Sterile Preparations

▶   Handling Hazardous Drugs

▶   Outsourcing Sterile Compounding Services

▶   Pharmacy-Prepared Ophthalmic Products

Products

▶   *Aseptic Compounding Technique: Learning and Mastering the Ritual* (Jordan ZT, ASHP, 2018)

▶   *Compounding Sterile Preparations*, 4th ed. (Buchanan EC, Forrey RA, Schneider PJ, ASHP, 2018)

▶   *Extended Stability for Parenteral Drugs*, 7th ed. (Simpson MC and Schaefer EG, ASHP, 2023)

▶   *Hazardous Drugs—Handling in Healthcare Settings: ASHP's Guide to USP Chapter <800>*

▶   Kienle PC, Eckel SF, Hansen KN. *Pharmacy Quick Reference Guide: Hazardous Drug Safety and Compliance with USP Chapter <800> in the Health System* (ASHP, October 15, 2022)

▶   *The Chapter <800> Answer Book* (Kienle PC, ASHP, 2017)

9.1-6   If a pharmacist has BPS board certification, do they need additional training?

Yes. Though the Board of Pharmacy Specialties Certified Sterile Compounding Pharmacist (BCSCP) certification[14] indicates the ability to successfully complete the didactic material, they also must be trained and be able to demonstrate successful completion of the same competencies you require for any compounder and demonstrate knowledge of your organizational policies and procedures.

9.1-7   If a technician has technician certification, do they need additional training?

Yes. The Pharmacy Technician Certification Board (PTCB) certification of CPhT indicates the ability to successfully complete a general pharmacy technician examination; it is not specific to sterile compounding. PTCB also has an additional technician certification for compounding sterile preparations.[15] Any pharmacy technician who mixes CSPs must be trained and be able to demonstrate successful completion of the same competencies you require for any compounder and demonstrate knowledge of your organizational policies and procedures.

9.1-8   If a technician has both a CPhT and the additional sterile compounding certification, do they need additional training?

Yes. Though the additional sterile compounding certification from the Pharmacy Technician Certification Board (PTCB) of Certified Compounded Sterile Preparation Technician (CSPT™)[15] indicates the ability to successfully complete the didactic material, they also must be trained and be able to demonstrate successful completion of the same competencies you require for any compounder and demonstrate knowledge of your organizational policies and procedures.

9.1-9   Our clerkship students are trained by the college prior to coming to hospital sites. Do they need additional training?

Yes. They also must be able to demonstrate successful completion of the same training and competencies you require for any compounder and demonstrate knowledge of your organizational policies and procedures if they will be compounding sterile preparations at your organization. Even if they have a document indicating successful completion of hand hygiene and garbing and aseptic processing (media fill, post media fill gloved fingertip test, and surface sample) at the college, it still must be repeated at your organization because those tests must reflect the facility conditions for your patients.

9.1-10 Who has to oversee the training and check off new personnel?

The oversight of this must be done by your designated person, but that person can delegate other qualified personnel to train and confirm competence of others.

9.1-11 Can a technician be the person who OKs a staff member's training, or does it have to be a pharmacist?

<797> does not restrict this to a pharmacist. Some states may require that this individual is a pharmacist.

9.1-12 Does training need to be documented?

Yes.

9.1-13 Does training documentation have to be written?

It can be written or electronic. Be sure it is retrievable because regulators and accreditation organization surveyors often ask to see these documents.

9.1-14 Do people who aren't compounding need training if they enter the IV room?

Yes. Anyone entering the sterile compounding suite or segregated compounding area (SCA) needs to be aware of restrictions. This includes administrative personnel, environmental services, surveyors, students, or anyone else. If they are not compounding or overseeing compounding, they don't necessarily need the same training as individuals who compound, but they still need to know what they may and may not do within the sterile compounding area. For example, a surveyor would not need institutional training but would need to be supervised while in the compounding area.

9.1-15 If pharmacists just check IVs but don't compound, do they need training?

It depends. If the pharmacists are in the sterile compounding area observing personnel who compound, they need to have the same competencies completed as those who routinely compound. However, pharmacists who may perform in-process checks (such as entering orders, viewing in-process photos or videos of steps in the compounding process, or other functions without entering the compounding area) may have competencies defined by organizational policy.

9.1-16 I'm the only pharmacist. Who has to train me?

A qualified person needs to train you. They could come to your site or you could attend an external program.

9.2 HAND HYGIENE

9.2-1 Is hand hygiene the same thing as hand washing?

Hand washing is a component of hand hygiene. See the CDC document on Hand Hygiene in Healthcare Settings[21] for complete information.

9.2-2 Where can I find a comprehensive description of hand hygiene?

See the CDC document on Hand Hygiene in Healthcare Settings[21] for complete information. The infection preventionist at your organization is a great source for this information.

9.2-3 Is soap and water OK to use for hand hygiene?

Yes. Hand washing with soap and water is required when compounding sterile preparations.

9.2-4 How often does a compounder need to demonstrate proper hand hygiene?

All compounders need to demonstrate competency initially. For requalification, it depends on the categories of CSPs compounded. Compounders who mix Category 1 or 2 CSPs must requalify at least every 6 months; those who mix Category 3 must requalify at least every 3 months. Designated persons who do not compound must requalify at least every 12 months.

9.2-5 Do people who are just checking IVs need to show competence in hand hygiene?

It depends. If the pharmacists are in the sterile compounding area observing personnel who compound they need to have the same competencies completed as those who routinely compound. However, pharmacists who may perform in-process checks (such as entering orders, viewing in-process photos or videos of steps in the compounding process, or other functions without entering the compounding area) may have competencies defined by organizational policy.

9.3 GARBING

9.3-1 How often does a compounder need to demonstrate proper garbing?

<797> requires garbing to be documented initially. To requalify, compounders who mix Category 1 or 2 CSPs must demonstrate competency at least every 6 months. Those who mix Category 3 CSPs must demonstrate competency at least every 3 months. Designated persons who do not compound must demonstrate competency at least every 12 months.

9.3-2 Do people who are just checking IVs need to demonstrate proper garbing procedures?

It depends. If the pharmacists are in the sterile compounding area observing personnel who compound they need to have the same competencies completed as those who routinely compound. However, pharmacists who may perform in-process checks (such as entering orders, viewing in-process photos or videos of steps in the compounding process, or other functions without entering the compounding area) may have competencies defined by organizational policy.

9.4 GLOVED FINGERTIP AND THUMB TEST AND SURFACE SAMPLING

9.4-1 What is the purpose of the gloved fingertip and thumb test?

There are two purposes:

▶ The initial and requalifying post-garbing gloved fingertip and thumb test is done to demonstrate that compounders can repeatedly garb without contaminating themselves.

▶ The initial and requalifying post-media fill gloved fingertip and thumb test is done after actual compounding to demonstrate the ability to maintain asepsis while compounding.

9.4-2 What type of media is used for a gloved fingertip and thumb test?

Use trypticase soy agar (TSA) that has been neutralized (e.g., with lecithin, polysorbate 80 [Tween 80]).

9.4-3 What is the proper procedure for doing a gloved fingertip and thumb test?

▶ Obtain one sampling device (e.g., plate) per hand.

▶ Label each sampling device with the compounder's name or initials, date and time of sampling, and right or left hand.

▶ Do **NOT** apply sterile 70% isopropyl alcohol or other solutions to the gloves immediately prior to sampling because this could cause false-negative results.

▶ Sample each hand by rolling fingers and thumb over the surface of the agar.

See Box 1 in <797> for complete information.

9.4-4 Where are the samples kept?

The media devices need to be incubated. The incubator temperature must be monitored and within the defined range.

9.4-5 How are the samples incubated?

▶ Store the media during incubation so condensation will not drip onto the surface. For example, store a media plate upside down.

▶ Incubate the samples at 30–35°C for at least 48 hours then at 20–25°C for at least 5 more days.

▶ Record the number of colony-forming units (CFUs) per hand. Total the number of CFUs on six plates (for the initial test) or both plates (for the requalifying test).

9.4-6 How and where is the initial gloved fingertip and thumb test done?

The person needs to follow your procedures, completing the full hand hygiene and garbing required for sterile compounding. Sample the person's glove inside a classified area (e.g., the anteroom) or the SCA. This needs to be repeated three separate times.

9.4-7 Can a person garb once and use three sets of plates at one time for the initial gloved fingertip and thumb test?

No. The purpose is to demonstrate the ability to repeatedly garb aseptically. The full hand hygiene and garbing must be done three separate times.

9.4-8 Do the three separate garbing sessions need to be done on the same day?

No. They can be done on the same day or on separate days. Three successful gloved fingertip and thumb tests must be completed before being allowed to compound independently.

9.4-9 How and where is the requalification gloved fingertip and thumb test done?

Two gloved fingertip and thumb tests must be done: one following hand hygiene and garbing and one as part of the aseptic processing (media fill, gloved fingertip test, surface sample) inside the PEC.

9.4-10 We use a compounding aseptic isolator (CAI). Does the gloved fingertip and thumb test need to be done inside the CAI?

Yes. The compounder needs to place sterile gloves over the gloves on the compounding isolator sleeves. The gloved fingertip and thumb test is done on those gloves. This applies to both the initial and the requalifying test because it needs to reflect the garbing and gloving procedure used at your organization.

9.4-11 How often is the requalification gloved fingertip and thumb test required?

Both the gloved fingertip test following garbing and the one as part of aseptic processing (media fill, gloved fingertip test, surface sample) must be successfully completed every 6 months for those mixing Category 1 and 2 CSPs and every 3 months for those mixing Category 3 CSPs. Designated persons who do not compound must demonstrate competency at least every 12 months.

9.4-12 Are three sets of media plates required for the requalification gloved fingertip and thumb test?

No. One set of plates—one plate for each hand—is required for the requalification gloved fingertip and thumb test following hand hygiene and garbing and another set of plates is required for part of aseptic processing requalification (media fill, gloved fingertip test, surface sample).

9.4-13 If someone passes two of the initial three gloved fingertip and thumb tests, do they have to repeat all three or just one?

They need to repeat all three (a total of six plates).

9.4-14 Is the training gloved fingertip and thumb test different from the one for requalification?

The procedure is the same. The location is different; the post-garbing test is done in the anteroom (if you have a cleanroom suite) or the SCA (if you have an SCA), and the post-media fill test is done in the PEC as part of aseptic processing evaluation (media fill, gloved fingertip test, surface sample). The action levels are different.

9.4-15 What does the *action level* mean?

The action level is the limit of growth—identified as CFUs—allowed. If the number of CFUs exceed the action level, some type of procedure is necessary to identify the reason and correct it.

9.4-16 Do the action level numbers apply to one hand or both hands?

Both hands must be tested. The action levels are based on the total CFUs detected (right hand plus left hand).

9.4-17 Do you need to sample both hands?

Yes. The four fingers and thumb of each hand needs to be sampled on a separate plate.

9.4-18 Can one plate be used for both hands?

No. The four fingers and thumb of each hand needs to be sampled on a separate plate.

9.4-19 What is the action level for the initial gloved fingertip and thumb test?

The action level for the initial post-garbing gloved fingertip and thumb test is anything greater than zero. This means that any CFUs detected on six plates (three tests of each hand) is unacceptable. The person needs to repeat the garbing and gloved fingertip and thumb test three times (for a total of six plates). The action level for the initial post-media fill gloved fingertip test is no more than three CFUs on both (not each) plate.

9.4-20 What is the action level for the requalification gloved fingertip and thumb test?

The action level for the requalifying post-garbing gloved fingertip and thumb test is zero. Only one set of plates is required for the requalifying tests. The action level for the requalifying post-media fill gloved fingertip and thumb test is no more than three CFUs on both (not each) plate.

9.4-21 Why must I have no growth on a gloved fingertip and thumb test when I'm learning, but when I'm really mixing IVs for patients, I can have some growth?

This seems counterintuitive but it's not because the two tests are for different purposes.

The *post-garbing glove fingertip and thumb test* is done to demonstrate compounders can repeatedly garb without contaminating themselves. It's done under controlled training conditions prior to actual compounding, so no growth on the media plates is allowed.

The *post-media fill gloved fingertip and thumb test* is done after actual compounding to demonstrate the ability to maintain asepsis while compounding. It's done as part of evaluating aseptic processing (media fill, followed by gloved fingertip and thumb test, followed by surface sample) in the PEC so is under conditions that reflect actual compounding.

9.4-22 If someone exceeds the action level, are they allowed to compound?

A new compounder needs to successfully complete the initial three gloved fingertip and thumb tests. <797> does not specifically state the action to take for compounding personnel completing the requalifying tests. However, the point of requalifying tests is to ensure competency. Your policy should address how this would be handled. In any case, results need to be documented and corrective actions (if any) described.

9.4-23 Do nurses who only mix immediate-use CSPs need to do a gloved fingertip and thumb test?

Personnel who mix only immediate-use CSPs are not required by <797> to complete a gloved fingertip and thumb or media fill test.

9.4-24 Do the nuclear medicine technologists need to do a gloved fingertip and thumb test?

USP General Chapter <825> Radiopharmaceuticals—Preparation, Compounding, Dispensing, and Repackaging[5] describes limitations of immediate use of sterile radiopharmaceuticals.

Note: This is a different definition than immediate use in <797>. Most hospital nuclear medicine department personnel only prepare sterile radiopharmaceuticals that meet the <825> immediate-use definition. If that is the case in your organization, the nuclear medicine technologists are not required to complete a gloved fingertip and thumb test by <825>. However, if more extensive compounding occurs in the nuclear medicine department, the gloved fingertip and thumb test and other requirements may need to be met. See <825> for full information. If the nuclear medicine technologists compound any sterile non-radiopharmaceuticals, they must comply with the requirements in <797>.

9.4-25 What is the purpose of surface sampling during personnel evaluation?

The physical tests - media fill, gloved fingertip and thumb testing, and surface sampling - are designed to ensure that the proper practices are used. The addition of a surface sample following the media fill and gloved fingertip sampling is clearly included in the 2023 revision of <797>. It reflects the ability to maintain an aseptic work space during compounding.

9.5 ASEPTIC TECHNIQUE

9.5-1 What is the definition of *aseptic technique*?

It is the process used to maintain asepsis during the compounding of sterile preparations. It encompasses proper garbing, maintenance of proper procedures, manipulations of components, and other procedural processes.

9.5-2 Is there a USP chapter about aseptic technique?

No, but refer to the information in ASHP's *Compounding Sterile Preparations*[28] and other compounding resources.

9.5-3 Does ASHP have any resources to teach aseptic technique?

Yes. There are a number of resources. See **Exhibit 9-1**. Remember that skills such as aseptic technique are best learned by reviewing didactic material, watching a skilled compounder, then providing return demonstration to the skilled compounder who can critique technique.

9.5-4 Is the aseptic technique nurses learn or the technique used in the operating room (OR) the same thing as the aseptic technique we need to use when compounding?

The principles are the same, but the procedures vary because the precision of sterile compounding differs from patient care activities.

9.5-5 What test is used to demonstrate competence in aseptic technique?

The media fill test simulates sterile compounding and is used to demonstrate the ability to aseptically manipulate the most complex CSP that a compounder could be expected to mix. The three physical tests—media fill, gloved fingertip and thumb test, and surface sampling—encompass the tests that evaluate aseptic manipulation.

9.6 MEDIA FILL TEST

9.6-1 What is the purpose of the media fill test?

The media fill test simulates sterile compounding and is used to demonstrate the ability to aseptically manipulate the most complex CSP that a compounder could be expected to mix.

9.6-2 How often does a media fill test have to be done?

Every sterile compounder needs to successfully complete a media fill test initially and at least every 6 months for those mixing Category 1 or 2 CSPs, and at least every 3 months for those mixing Category 3 CSPs. Personnel who oversee compounding but who do not compound need to successfully complete a media fill at least every 12 months.

9.6-3 How do I design a media fill test?

Compounders need to simulate the most complex CSP that they would mix. It may be the number of manipulations, the need to achieve sterility rather than only maintain sterility, use of specific equipment, or other factors that increase the complexity of the CSPs mixed at your site.

9.6-4 Can I use a commercially available kit for a media fill test?

Yes, if it mimics the most complex CSP you mix.

9.6-5 What kind of media and devices are used for a media fill test?

Soybean-casein digest media is used. The laboratory you use can provide you with sources. The devices are dependent on the most complex CSP you mix. It may be IV bags and vials. It may include using an automated compounder, ambulatory infusion pump, or other container or device. Mimic the components and devices you use.

9.6-6 We use a CAI. Do we still need to do a media fill test?

Yes. The media fill test is required for anyone who compounds CSPs in a cleanroom or segregated compounding area.

9.6-7 Does everyone on staff need to do the same media fill test?

Not necessarily, unless required by your state or organizational policy. However, consider your staffing patterns and work needs. The media fill test needs to mimic the most complex CSP a compounder would be asked to prepare.

9.6-8 What is the proper procedure for doing a media fill test?

The procedure is dependent on the media fill test you use. Commercially available kits have instructions that meet the components in the kit. If you create your own, develop a procedure that mimics the manipulations necessary to mix the most complex CSP you prepare.

9.6-9 If I mix nonsterile-to-sterile preparations, can I use purchased soybean-casein digest media?

If you mix nonsterile-to-sterile CSPs, you need to start with nonsterile soybean-casein digest powder.

9.6-10 Can I start with nonsterile media and mix it myself?

If you are simulating nonsterile-to-sterile preparations, you need to do that, and to include at least one positive control to show growth promotion capability. See the section in *USP General Chapter <71> Sterility Tests* that details Culture Media and Incubation Temperatures, Growth Promotion Test of Aerobes, Anaerobes, and Fungi.[29]

9.6-11 Is there specific information I need to keep concerning the media used?

You need to keep the lot-specific Certificate of Analysis (CoA) that says it will support the growth of microorganisms.

9.6-12 Do I need an incubator?

Yes. The tests need to be incubated. Pharmacy doesn't necessarily need to have the incubator in the department. Some organizations have the microbiology laboratory incubate the tests. If you do have an incubator, it cannot be inside the sterile compounding area.

9.6-13 Can I use a mannitol warmer to incubate the media fill tests?

No. Most mannitol warmers are not sufficiently controlled or calibrated to maintain the required incubation temperatures.

9.6-14 At what temperature and for how long do the media fill tests need to be incubated?

Incubate them for 7 days at 20–25°C, then for an additional 7 days at 30–35°C.

9.6-15 Is there an action level for media fill tests?

The media fill test is pass/fail. A negative test is good; no turbidity or color change is present after incubation. A failed test is one where turbidity or other growth occurs prior to the end of the 14-day incubation period.

9.6-16 Where is the initial media fill test done?

The media fill test simulates the most complex CSP you mix. It is done inside the PEC.

9.6-17 Where is the requalification media fill test done?

The media fill test simulates the most complex CSP you mix. It is done inside the PEC.

9.6-18 What should be documented?

Compounder's name, date of the test, media used (manufacturer, lot number, expiry), incubation location and temperature records, results of the test, who read the results, and who documented the results.

9.6-19 Do nurses who only mix immediate-use CSPs need to do a media fill test?

Personnel who mix only immediate-use CSPs are not required by <797> to complete a gloved fingertip or media fill test.

9.6-20 Do the nuclear medicine technologists need to do a media fill test?

<825> describes limitations of immediate use of sterile radiopharmaceuticals.

Note: This is a different definition than immediate use in <797>. Most hospital nuclear medicine department personnel only compound sterile radiopharmaceuticals that meet the <825> immediate-use definition. If that is the case in your organization, the nuclear medicine technologists are not required to complete a media fill test by <825>. However, if more extensive compounding occurs in the nuclear medicine department, the media fill test and other requirements may need to be met. See <825>[5] for full information. If the nuclear medicine technologists compound any sterile nonradiopharmaceuticals, they must comply with the requirements in <797>.

9.7 REQUALIFICATION

9.7-1 How often does retraining need to occur?

Successful completion of post-garbing gloved fingertip and thumb test and aseptic processing (media fill, gloved fingertip and thumb test, surface sample) must occur at least every 6 months for compounders who mix Category 1 or 2 CSPs and at least every 3 months for those who mix Category 3 CSPs. Designated persons who do not compound must demonstrate competency at least every 12 months. Other core competencies must be documented at least every 12 months, but consider some—such as visual observation of hand hygiene and garbing—more frequently.

9.7-2 If someone has been on leave, or has not compounded for a while, do they need to demonstrate competence before they can compound?

If the time has elapsed since they have qualified (depending on the categories of CSPs they mix and your organizational policy), they must requalify.

9.7-3 Do I need to document the requalification?

Yes.

9.7-4 Who needs to keep the records for training and requalification? Pharmacy? Human Resources? The individual?

The organization needs to maintain the documented competence in the employee's human resource records. It is up to the organization concerning the storage, but be sure that the records are retrievable because an inspector or surveyor could ask for them.

STERILE PRODUCTS AND SUPPLIES *10*

10.1 GENERAL INFORMATION

10.1-1 What is the difference between the terms *products* and *preparations*?

Products are conventionally manufactured items. *Preparations* are compounded. Note that the FDA uses the term *products* for items compounded by an outsourcing facility.

10.1-2 What are conventionally manufactured products?

Conventionally manufactured products are those produced by pharmaceutical manufacturers. This differs from compounds, which can be provided by pharmacies (503A entities) or by FDA-registered outsourcing facilities (503B entities).

10.1-3 Does <797> deal with manufactured products? I thought it was only about compounded sterile preparations.

<797> is a comprehensive standard about sterile compounding. Conventionally manufactured products (e.g., intravenous [IV] bags, injection vials) are the key components of compounded sterile preparations (CSPs).

10.1-4 What are considered components of a CSP?

Components include the *ingredients* (i.e., drug, diluent, excipient), the *containers* (e.g., bags, syringes, vials) in which CSPs are placed, and the *closure-system* (e.g., cap) used.

10.2 USE OF NONSTERILE STARTING COMPONENTS

10.2-1 What is an API?

An API—active pharmaceutical ingredient—is defined by <797> as "any substance or mixture of substances intended to be used in the compounding of a preparation, thereby becoming the active ingredient in that preparation and furnishing pharmacological activity or other direct effect in the diagnosis, cure, mitigation, treatment, or prevention of disease in humans and animals or affecting the structure and function of the body."[3] It's informally referred to as *bulk drug substance, bulk powder,* or *raw material.*

DOI 10.37573/9781585287260.010

10.2-2 Do all components need to be marked *USP* or *NF*?

APIs must be obtained from a supplier that is registered with the FDA, so they will be marked *United States Pharmacopeia (USP)* or *National Formulary (NF)* if a monograph exists for the ingredient. Refer to FDA's guidance documents on compounding with bulk substances for more information.

10.2-3 Why do I have to use an API that's from an FDA-registered supplier?

It's a federal regulation. Section 503A of the Federal Food, Drug, and Cosmetic Act requires bulk drug substances to be manufactured by an establishment registered with the FDA.[30]

10.2-4 I need to use an excipient that doesn't have a *USP* or *NF* monograph. Where do I get it?

Obtain it from an FDA-registered supplier if you can. If you can't, a designated person needs to ensure that it is of appropriate quality and suitable for use.

10.2-5 How do I know the quality of the component?

You need a lot-specific Certificate of Analysis (CoA) for any component that is not a commercial drug. That document tells you the quality standards and other information related to the component.

10.2-6 Is water a component?

Yes. Use *sterile water for injection* or *sterile water for irrigation* (as appropriate for the dosage form) when mixing CSPs requiring water.[31]

10.2-7 I have some chemicals marked ACS. Are they OK to use?

Chemicals may be marked ACS (American Chemical Society), but that doesn't necessarily mean they are safe to use. They haven't been tested for pharmaceutical use in humans or animals.

10.2-8 I have a shelf full of old chemicals. Many are marked *USP* or *NF*. Are they OK to use?

If they are marked with an expiration date and that date has not yet passed, they are OK to use as long as they have been stored properly, and the container and API appear undamaged. If they don't have an expiration date and you received them more than 1 year ago (or you can't tell when they were received), they need to be appropriately discarded.

10.2-9 If I received a chemical without an expiration date, do I need to assign a date?

Yes. Record the date of receipt, mark the date of receipt on the container, assign an expiration date that doesn't exceed 1 year from the date of receipt, and mark the expiry on the container.

10.2-10 Can I start the 1-year expiry from the date I open the jar?

No. It has to be a maximum of 1 year from the date you received it.

10.2-11 The alum we use has a manufacturer's expiration date. Do I need to discard it after 1 year?

No. You can use the manufacturer-assigned expiry as long as you are confident that it has been stored properly and the ingredient, container, and closure (e.g., lid) are not compromised.

FACILITY DESIGN, ENGINEERING CONTROLS, AND EQUIPMENT 11

11.1 GENERAL FACILITY DESIGN INFORMATION

11.1-1 What are the minimum facility requirements for compounding sterile preparations?

CSPs must be compounded in an area that is specifically designated for sterile compounding and meets the requirements in <797>. The surfaces in the area need to be able to withstand the cleaning and sanitizing agents required following compounding. The floor cannot be carpeted. Temperature must be controlled to meet manufacturers' requirements for drug storage and for the comfort of personnel. Your state regulations may have additional requirements.

11.1-2 Are there different minimum facility requirements for compounding hazardous sterile preparations?

Yes. Hazardous drugs (HDs) must be compounded in a room that is separate from compounding of non-HDs. The room must have fixed walls, be negative pressure, be vented to the outside, and have the appropriate number of air changes per hour (ACPH). Sterile compounding anterooms and buffer rooms require at least 30 ACPH. See <800>[4] and *The Chapter <800> Answer Book*[9] for more information.

11.1-3 What engineering controls are required by <797>?

<797> requires a primary engineering control (PEC), commonly called a *hood*, and a secondary engineering control (SEC), the room in which the hood resides. (There is a special situation for compounding allergen extracts, which has a different requirement. See Section 11.14.)

11.1-4 Is an engineering control and a PEC the same thing?

A PEC, commonly called a *hood*, is a type of engineering control. The room in which the hood is placed is called an *SEC*.

11.1-5 What does *classified* mean?

Classified devices or rooms mean that they meet the requirements of the International Organization for Standardization (ISO) standard 14644-1 for classification of air cleanliness for cleanrooms and associated controlled environments, where

DOI 10.37573/9781585287260.011

the number of particles allowed is under the limit for that designation. PECs must be ISO 5 or better. (*Better* means fewer particles, which is a lower ISO number.) Buffer rooms must be ISO 7 or better. Anterooms must be ISO 7 or better if they open into a negative buffer room but can be ISO 8 (or better) if they open into only positive buffer rooms. Segregated compounding areas (SCAs) or containment segregated compounding areas (C-SCAs) are not required to be ISO classified.

11.1-6 Does the sterile compounding area need to be a separate room?

A cleanroom suite needs to have at least two separate rooms (anteroom and buffer room). An SCA should be a separate room but may be a separate area that is defined by a visible perimeter. A C-SCA must be a separate room.

A combined ante/buffer room was permitted in the 2008 version of <797> but does not meet the requirement for a cleanroom suite. It may meet the requirement of an SCA.

11.1-7 Can noncompounding activities occur in the compounding area?

No.

11.1-8 Is it OK to use part of the intravenous (IV) room for office-related space, like order entry and processing?

No. Anterooms, buffer rooms, and SCAs need to be restricted to activities related to sterile compounding.

11.1-9 Is there a restriction concerning who can enter the IV room?

Only authorized personnel may enter the area, but that definition is up to you and needs to be described in your policies and procedures.

11.1-10 How much space is necessary for compounding?

That is based on your practice and needs. Be sure to allow space for any equipment you use for compounding. In many states, the state board of pharmacy regulations dictates a minimum area or linear square feet of counter space.

11.1-11 Can I use plastic curtains or drapes to define the compounding area?

No, not in cleanroom suites. <797> does not prohibit this in SCAs, but it's not a good idea. Dividers made of these materials are very difficult to keep clean. <800> required fixed walls, so plastic curtains or drapes are not allowed for a HD compounding area.

11.1-12 Does the hood need to be on emergency power?

<797> doesn't specify this but some accreditation organizations standards do. In any case, it is a good idea.

11.1-13 Can I use the same compounding room for both nonhazardous and hazardous sterile compounding?

No. If you compound both nonhazardous and the National Institute for Occupational Safety and Health (NIOSH) Table 1 antineoplastic CSPs,[19] you need a separate room for each type of sterile compounding. Note that <800> allows you to entity-exempt some nonantineoplastic drugs on the NIOSH list of HDs if you perform an Assessment of Risk and identity and implement alternative strategies for containment and work practices. See <800>[4] and *The Chapter <800> Answer Book*[9] for details about hazardous compounding.

The 2008 version of <797> allowed placement of a containment primary engineering control (BSC or CACI) in a positive buffer room, as long as only a low volume of antineoplastics were mixed. This is not permitted by <800> and is no longer permitted by <797>.

11.1-14 Do I need a separate room for receiving sterile products?

No. There is no requirement in <797> for receiving areas. However, do not allow totes or other external packages to be received or opened in your sterile compounding rooms; they have been in dirty areas and could contaminate your sterile compounding area.

11.1-15 What type of sink do I need, and where should it be placed?

Your sink needs to be easily accessible to your compounding area. Be sure your sink is big enough and deep enough so you can wash your hands and arms up to your elbows without splashing adjacent counters. Stainless steel is best; ceramic sinks are prone to chipping so they become an infection control risk. Ideally, have a sink dedicated for compounding.

11.1-16 Should the sink be next to the hood?

Sinks are not permitted in the buffer room. The placement of the sink and the garbing practices you use need to be designed to work efficiently and safely together. Your sink needs to be at least 1 meter away from the hood in an SCA.

11.1-17 Why does a sink need to be at least 1 meter away from the hood?

It has to be at least 1 meter away from the hood to minimize the chance of microbial contamination from splashing.

11.1-18 Should the garb storage be adjacent to the sink?

No, but it needs to be close enough to efficiently garb. Placing garb right next to the sink could allow splashing and contamination of the garb.

11.1-19 Are there any temperature or humidity requirements for the sterile compounding area?

The temperature of the storage area for compounding components must be maintained based on the requirement of the CSPs or the components. Also consider the comfort of the compounders. <797> recommends a temperature not greater than 20° for the comfort of garbed compounders. Your relative humidity should be below 60%.

Whatever temperature range and humidity is acceptable must be defined in your policies and must be monitored and recorded daily (when the pharmacy is open, unless required daily by your state). It can be recorded on a log or by a continuous monitoring device; the information must be retrievable. Staff members need to know what to do if the temperature or humidity is out of range. Thermometers and humidity monitoring devices must be calibrated or verified at least every 12 months or as required by the manufacturer.

11.1-20 If the humidity is low, should I put in a humidifier?

No. Don't add any water sources like this to the area. There is no need to adjust for low humidity in compounding areas.

11.1-21 What are the minimum air changes per hour required by <797>?

ISO 7 areas require at least 30 ACPH. ISO 8 areas require at least 20 ACPH.

Area	Minimum ACPH
Anteroom that opens only into a positive buffer room(s)	20
Anteroom that opens into any negative buffer room	30
Positive pressure buffer room	30
Negative pressure buffer room	30

Up to 15 ACPH may come from a PEC that is vented back into the room. At least 15 must come from the air handling system.

11.1-22 Can I depend on any type of PEC to be able to contribute 15 ACPH?

No. Laminar airflow workbenches (LAFWs), compounding aseptic isolators (CAIs), biological safety cabinets (BSCs), and containment ventilated enclosures (CVEs) that are vented into the room may contribute up to 15 ACPH. Compounding aseptic containment isolators (CACIs) and BSCs that are externally vented cannot contribute to the ACPH total. Your certifier needs to indicate the source and total ACPH on your certification report.

11.1-23 Because <797> lists a minimum number of ACPH, is there any need to use a higher number?

Yes. Don't design for the minimum, because you will see changes over time. The number of ACPH needed to maintain the environment depends on the number of people in the room and the activities performed. As the high efficiency particulate air (HEPA) filters in the ceiling age, they become less efficient and don't allow as much air to pass through them. If your room has 30 ACPH when new, you will see a decrease as the room is used.

11.1-24 How many ACPH are required for an SCA?

An SCA used for nonhazardous drugs does not have a required ACPH. A containment SCA used for HDs must have at least 12 ACPH.

11.1-25 Where should the gauges be for the temperature, humidity, and pressure?

There is no specific information in <797> but consider placing them outside the sterile compounding area. That way, you don't have to enter the room to read the information.

11.1-26 What kind of finishes do I need to use for floors, walls, and ceilings?

Surfaces of ceilings, walls, floors, fixtures, shelving, counters, and cabinets in a cleanroom suite must be smooth, impervious, free from cracks and crevices, non-shedding, and cleanable. An SCA should have these same characteristics.

11.1-27 What documents should my certifier reference on certification reports?

Your certifier should use the Controlled Environment Testing Association's (CETA) certification guide for sterile compounding facilities[32] or a document that provides the information required by <797>.

11.1-28 Is there a way to summarize the key certification results?

If your certifier does not provide a summary sheet, consider using the summary in Exhibit 13-1.

11.2 STORAGE AREAS

11.2-1 I have heard that cardboard isn't allowed in the compounding area. Is that true?

No shipping cartons, corrugated cardboard, or uncoated cardboard is allowed in a cleanroom suite or SCA. Most accreditation organizations expect the facility to do a risk assessment concerning placement of cardboard. If this applies to your organization, be sure to designate the compounding areas as clean areas and restrict external shipping containers and corrugated cardboard from the area.

11.2-2 Can shipping boxes be taken into the compounding area?

No. Accreditation organizations often require the organization to do a risk assessment for storage of cardboard. Because any compounding area should be designated as a clean area, no external shipping containers or corrugated cardboard should be allowed in the sterile compounding area.

11.2-3 IV bags and other supplies used for compounding come in cardboard boxes. What is the best way to store these?

When the supplies need to be moved into the compounding area, remove them from the cardboard outside the area and place them in labeled plastic bins. If the supplies were not protected by plastic, you may need to wipe them with a suitable agent prior to placement in the bins.

11.2-4 Do storage rooms require a specific ACPH?

<797> does not have a requirement for ACPH in storage areas. <800> has a requirement of 12 ACPH for HD storage areas.

11.2-5 Is it OK to store supplies on the floor?

No. Do not place components or other supplies directly on the floor.

11.3 PRIMARY ENGINEERING CONTROLS

11.3-1 What should I look for when buying a hood?

The PEC, commonly called a *hood,* is a sophisticated engineering control used for sterile compounding. It is not the same as a fume hood or a glove box, so those terms should not be used to describe the device required for sterile compounding. A number of manufacturers make PECs designed for sterile compounding. All must maintain unidirectional flow of air and must meet ISO 5 requirements for air quality. See <797> for complete requirements.[3]

11.3-2 How often do hoods for sterile compounding have to be certified?

Hood must be certified upon commissioning (when you first use it), at least every 6 months, and whenever it is moved or serviced.

11.3-3 Is there an industry guidance for testing/certification of a hood?

Yes. CETA publishes certification guides.[32] The PEC needs to meet the minimum requirements of the applicable guide.

11.3-4 Is it OK to turn off the hood when we aren't using it?

No. The hood must remain powered on except for servicing or moving.

11.3-5 Can I use the same device for both nonhazardous and chemo sterile compounding?

If you compound both nonhazardous and NIOSH Table 1 antineoplastic CSPs, you need a separate device for each type of sterile compounding. (<800> allows occasional compounding of nonhazardous CSP in a BSC or CACI in a negative pressure buffer room or C-SCA, but because any component or CSP compounded in that space needs to be considered potentially contaminated and must be labeled with personal protective equipment precautions, it is not a practical process.) Note that <800> allows you to entity-exempt some drugs on the NIOSH list (though not any that are API or Table 1 antineoplastics that need to be manipulated) if you perform an Assessment of Risk and identity and implement alternative strategies for containment and work practices. See <800>[4] and *The Chapter <800> Answer Book*[9] for details about hazardous compounding.

11.3-6 Is a robot a PEC?

Yes, if it functions as a device in which CSPs are mixed. The robot needs to meet the definition of the specific type of PEC it is designed to be.

11.3-7 How many people can work in one hood?

It should be limited to one. Some organizations allow two people to work in 8-foot hoods, but there must be a clear division between the workspace. Consider the medication safety issues that can present if more than one person works in a hood. The Institute for Safe Medication Practices' (ISMP) *Guidelines for Safe Preparation of Compounded Sterile Preparations*[33] provides a review of safety considerations.

11.3-8 Does the pressure need to be documented every day for the space in the CAI?

<797> does not require that documentation but the manufacturer of your CAI or CACI may recommend it.

11.3-9 Are CAIs primary or secondary engineering controls?

CAIs are the primary control. A secondary engineering control is the buffer room or segregated compounding area in which the CAI is placed.

11.3-10 Does a CAI need to be in a cleanroom suite?

To use the full BUDs allowed by <797>, the CAI needs to be in the buffer room of a cleanroom suite. If it is not in the buffer room, it can be the PEC in an SCA.

11.3-11 We have a system that includes a camera inside the hood. Is this OK?

Yes, as long as the PEC meets certification requirements under dynamic conditions.

11.3-12 We have a system that includes a scale inside the hood. Is this OK?

Yes, as long as the PEC meets certification requirements under dynamic conditions.

11.3-13 We have a system that includes a touchscreen monitor inside the hood. Is this OK?

Yes, as long as the PEC meets certification requirements under dynamic conditions.

11.4 SECONDARY ENGINEERING CONTROLS— GENERAL INFORMATION

11.4-1 What is a secondary engineering control (SEC)?

The SEC is the room in which CSPs are mixed. A cleanroom suite has an anteroom and at least one buffer room. A SCA is a type of secondary engineering control that is acceptable but requires use of short BUDs.

11.4-2 Are modular rooms OK to have?

SCAs can be either stick built or modular. They have the same facility requirements.

11.4-3 What kind of things do I need to be sure our architects, facility department, and contractor need to consider when designing our IV room?

Your sterile compounding area needs to be designed to meet at least the minimum physical facility issues and needs to reflect your workflow. What works at one place may not be appropriate for another place.

Be sure to consider the following:

▶ The space you need for the scope of practice—Be sure to know the potential for future expansion plans when the hospital's patient mix changes significantly (either by volume or specific services).

▶ The number of people you generally have in each room—The ACPH are minimum requirements and often need to be higher when more than one person is in the room.

▶ The air handling system capacity—Most compliant sterile compounding areas have a dedicated air handler.

▶ Temperature and humidity requirements of the rooms

▶ The pressure requirements of the rooms (anteroom, positive pressure buffer room for nonhazardous CSPs, negative pressure room for antineoplastic CSPs)—If you have other sophisticated needs (e.g., gene therapy), be sure to design appropriate space.

▶ The surfaces and finishes of the floors, walls, and ceilings

▶ Placement and number of ceiling HEPA filters

▶ Installation of ports to allow your certifier to test the integrity of the ceiling HEPA filters

▶ Low air returns and exhausts

▶ Exhausts for negative pressure rooms

▶ Space for solutions and equipment used for cleaning

▶ PEC placement

▶ Placement of sink

▶ Placement of plumbed eye wash

- ▸ Placement and types of doors separating the rooms
- ▸ Use of flush-mounted, cleanable sprinkler heads
- ▸ Placement of shelving
- ▸ Airtight sealing with cleanroom-compliant caulk for housings of light fixtures, mirrors, electrical outlets, computer drops, etc.
- ▸ Solid mobile stainless steel shelving and tables
- ▸ Placement and type of refrigerators

As you develop designs of the room, consider taping off the room size and hood and other equipment placement and walking through the area to ensure the space is adequate for your workflow.

11.4-4 Do all surfaces have to be stainless steel?

No, but stainless steel is a good choice because it is durable and will withstand the decontamination and cleaning needed.

11.4-5 Is every sterile compounding room an SEC?

An SEC must meet the facility requirements listed in <797>.

11.4-6 Is an SEC positive or negative pressure, or can it be neutral pressure?

In a cleanroom suite, the anteroom must be positive to the adjacent space. A buffer room used for nonhazardous CSPs must be positive to the anteroom. A buffer room used for mixing antineoplastic NIOSH Table 1 antineoplastic CSPs[19] must be negative to the anteroom. An SCA can be neutral/normal pressure. A C-SCA must be negative to the adjacent space.

11.4-7 Is a chemo room an SEC?

Yes. NIOSH Table 1 antineoplastics ("chemo") need to be mixed in a room with at least these characteristics:

- ▸ Room with fixed walls that is separate from nonhazardous compounding
- ▸ Negative pressure between 0.010″ to 0.030″ wc
- ▸ Vented to the outside
- ▸ At least 12 ACPH for a C-SCA and at least 30 ACPH for a negative pressure buffer room

11.4-8 How big should an SEC be?

<797> does not define this; your state board may. It needs to be big enough to adequately handle the compounding you do.

11.4-9 Is it OK to use the SEC for order entry if it's related to sterile compounding?

No. The SEC should be restricted to the activities directly related to sterile compounding.

11.4-10 Can the SEC be used to store drugs, IV solutions, and supplies?

Yes, but it should not be the general storage area. Remember that all supplies need to be cleaned at least every month, so anything inside the anteroom or buffer room needs to be removed for monthly cleaning.

11.4-11 Can I put shelving in my sterile compounding area?

Yes, as long as the room meets certification requirements under dynamic conditions.

11.4-12 Can I put a refrigerator in my sterile compounding area?

Yes, as long as the room meets certification requirements under dynamic conditions. Pass-through refrigerators are not allowed in negative rooms. Refrigerators are environmental challenges and must be meticulously maintained.

11.4-13 Can I put a printer in my sterile compounding area?

Yes, as long as the room meets certification requirements under dynamic conditions.

11.4-14 How do I calculate room air change rates?

ACPHs are calculated by using the room volume (length × width × height) and dividing it into the cubic feet of air per minute. (ACPH = CFM × 60/room volume.)

11.4-15 Do the monitors for temperature, humidity, and pressure have to be inside the IV room?

No. They may be located inside the sterile compounding room but they add to the number of pieces of equipment that must be cleaned daily. Also consider the impact on the room if the monitors need servicing or replacement. It may be more efficient and present fewer potential challenges if the monitors are located outside of the cleanroom.

11.4-16 What is the distinction between the dirty and clean side of an SEC?

The *dirty side* of the anteroom is where you enter it from the uncontrolled (not ISO-classified) area. The *clean side* is where final garbing occurs. The garbing functions that occur in either side needs to be dependent on the placement of your sink and needs to be defined in your policies and procedures. (See Section 9.3 on garbing.)

11.5 ANTEROOMS

11.5-1 What is an anteroom?

The anteroom is a transition room that is part of the sterile compounding suite. It is a room where garbing occurs. It needs to be marked with a line of demarcation that separates the dirty side (the side you walk into) from the clean side (where gowns and gloves are donned). In most facilities, the sink is on the clean side of the anteroom. The doors to the buffer rooms are on the clean side of the anteroom.

11.5-2 What are the physical requirements for an anteroom?

The anteroom needs to be a separate room, positive pressure (at least 0.020″ wc more positive than the adjacent space that is not part of the cleanroom suite), with at least ISO 8 air quality (at least ISO 7 if it opens into any negative space), and have the appropriate finishes on the floors, walls, and ceilings.

11.5-3 Does every sterile compounding room need an anteroom?

Every sterile compounding suite requires an anteroom. An SCA, C-SCA, or allergenic extracts compounding area (AECA) does not necessarily have to have anterooms but does need space within the area to complete garbing.

11.5-4 Is an anteroom positive or negative pressure, or can it be neutral pressure?

An anteroom must be *positive* pressure to the non-classified workspace adjacent to it. It is designed with positive pressure to control antimicrobial and other particle contamination from entering the compounding suite.

11.5-5 Because our chemo room is negative pressure, does the anteroom for that need to be negative pressure?

No. The anteroom is always *positive* pressure. That protects the compounding suite from contamination.

11.5-6 Is more than one anteroom required if we have a positive and a negative buffer room?

One anteroom can serve both negative and positive buffer rooms.

11.5-7 How big should an anteroom be?

<797> does not define this but your state board may. It needs to be big enough to adequately handle the garbing and hand hygiene activities for the compounding you do.

11.5-8 Is there a minimum square footage requirement?

<797> does not define this, but your state board may.

11.5-9 Is there a minimum square footage requirement based on the number of people in the room?

<797> does not define this, but your state board may.

11.5-10 Is it OK to use the anteroom for order entry if it's related to sterile compounding?

The anteroom should be restricted to the garbing and hand hygiene processes. The more activities that occur in the anteroom, the more risk of microbial and other contamination.

11.5-11 Can the anteroom have a pneumatic tube?

No. That would be a significant infection control risk.

11.5-12 Can the anteroom be used to store drugs, IV solutions, and supplies?

It can but limit the amount of stock. Remember that all shelving must be cleaned monthly. All products and supplies located in the anteroom, buffer room, or within the perimeter around a PEC in an SCA must have been cleaned at least monthly.

11.5-13 Can the anteroom have shelves?

Yes, if necessary, to store the products and supplies you store in the area. Consider use of solid (not wire) shelves to make cleaning easier.

11.5-14 What is the distinction between the dirty and clean side of an anteroom?

The *dirty side* is the side you enter from. The *clean side* is the side closest to the entrances to the buffer rooms.

11.5-15 What is the line of demarcation in the anteroom?

The line of demarcation separates the area in which you enter (dirty side) from the area where final garbing takes place (clean side).

11.5-16 What is the distinction between a wet and dry anteroom?

Some facilities have a more structured process for garbing and have separate rooms in which garbing takes place. The *wet* anteroom contains the sink. The *dry* anteroom does not. This is not a required design but can be used to support more controlled garbing. It is similar to the process used in pharmaceutical manufacturing facilities.

11.5-17 Can the anteroom have a sink?

Yes. Most facilities have the sink on the clean side of the anteroom, which was the generally accepted design in previous versions of <797>.

11.5-18 Does the anteroom have to have a sink?

A sink needs to be available for sterile compounding hand hygiene. Most facilities have the sink on the clean side of the anteroom, but some more structured designs have separate anterooms (wet and dry anterooms). All organizations need to design their policies and procedures to support the design of the area.

11.5-19 My SCA is ISO 7. Does it need an anteroom?

You need an anteroom with an attached buffer room to use the full BUDs. If you have an SCA or C-SCA, an anteroom is not required but the BUDs are limited to those for Category 1 CSPs.

11.5-20 If I put a CAI in the anteroom, is that considered a cleanroom suite?

No. To be a cleanroom suite, your PEC needs to be in a buffer room that is entered from a separate anteroom.

11.5-21 What kind of finishes should be used for the floor, walls, and ceiling of an anteroom?

The finishes of an anteroom are the same as a buffer room: they must be "smooth, impervious, free from cracks and crevices, and nonshedding."[3]

11.5-22 Is it OK to separate the sides of an anteroom by putting tape on the floor?

No. The tape will loosen over time and create a surface to attract particles and other contamination. Install a permanent line, such as using a different color flooring.

11.6 PRESTERILIZATION AREA FOR WEIGHING POWDERS

11.6-1 Where should powders be weighed for preparation of sterile CSPs?

Presterilization procedures for Category 2 or 3 CSPs, including weighing and mixing, must be performed in a PEC in a room that is ISO 8 or cleaner. Unless this is done in a room separate from the anteroom or buffer room used for compounding CSPs, you need to weigh and handle powders only when no sterile compounding is occurring. The room must be able to maintain ISO Class 8 while the powder-weighing is occurring.

Ideally, you should have a separate room (often part of the cleanroom suite) that contains a PEC dedicated for this purpose, such as a containment ventilated enclosure (CVE) (e.g., a powder containment hood). The weighing and mixing would occur there and then transported in a closed container into the buffer room for filtration (when applicable), compounding, and packaging. Personnel must be garbed the same as when working in an ISO 5 PEC.

11.6-2 Do I need a separate area for weighing powders if I never mix CSPs from nonsterile ingredients?

No. Most organizations mix CSPs only from sterile components. If this is the case, there is no need for a separate weighing room.

11.7 CLEANROOM SUITES

11.7-1 What are the minimum room requirements for a cleanroom suite?

A compounding suite must minimally contain a positive pressure anteroom and at least one buffer room (positive pressure for nonhazardous drugs or negative pressure for HDs).

11.7-2 What does a cleanroom suite have that an SCA doesn't have?

An SCA is not required to have HEPA-filtered ceiling air nor is it required to be ISO classified.

11.7-3 I have a combined ante/buffer room. Is this a cleanroom suite?

No. A cleanroom suite must contain a minimum of two rooms: an anteroom and at least one buffer room. The combined ante/buffer room allowed in the 2008 version of <797> is no longer considered a cleanroom. It may meet the requirement of an SCA.

11.7-4 What is the ISO requirement for a cleanroom suite?

The buffer rooms need to be at least ISO 7. The anteroom needs to be at least ISO 7 if it opens into any negative room and must be at least ISO 8 if it opens into only positive pressure buffer rooms.

11.7-5 Are ceiling HEPA filters required?

Yes. The air entering the cleanroom suite (both the anterooms and buffer rooms) must come from HEPA filters placed in the ceiling of the room.

11.7-6 I have HEPA filters in the ceiling and the air returns about a foot down from the ceiling. Is this OK?

Probably not. The air returns/exhausts should be low on the wall to allow the HEPA-filtered air to sweep throughout the room. If the air returns are not low on the walls, your certifier needs to do a smoke study of the room to demonstrate that air is not stagnating in any area.

11.7-7 Does a cleanroom suite require an isolator?

A cleanroom suite requires any acceptable PEC allowed by <797>: a laminar air flow system (e.g., LAFW, BSC), a restricted access barrier system (RABS) (e.g., CAI, CACI), or a pharmaceutical isolator. A RABS or pharmaceutical isolator can be used in a cleanroom suite but it is not the only acceptable PEC.

11.7-8 I have a combined anteroom/buffer room that is ISO 7. I heard this is no longer allowed in new <797>. Is this true?

That is true; it is not a cleanroom. It may meet the requirement of an SCA.

11.7-9 Where does the sink need to be placed in a cleanroom suite?

The sink may be placed inside (on the clean or dirty side) or outside the anteroom in a cleanroom suite. In an SCA, the sink may be inside the SCA (but at least 1 meter from the PEC) or in close proximity.

11.7-10 Are there separate requirements for a cleanroom suite used for chemo?

Yes. The negative buffer room used for HDs must have 4 minimum criteria:

▶ Room with fixed walls that is separate from nonhazardous compounding
▶ Negative pressure between 0.010″ to 0.030″ wc negative to adjacent space
▶ Vented to the outside
▶ At least 30 ACPH (12 ACPH is acceptable in a C-SCA)

See <800>[4] and *The Chapter <800> Answer Book*[9] for more information.

11.7-11 Can the air conditioning be turned off in the cleanroom suite when it's not in use?

No.

11.7-12 Can the number of air changes per hour be lowered when the cleanroom suite is not in use?

No.

11.7-13 Are portable HEPA filters OK to use?

They cannot be the only source of HEPA-filtered air. The air handing system must provide the minimum number of ACPHs. If used, a portable HEPA filter needs to be certified as leak-free.

11.7-14 How many people can work in a cleanroom suite?

That is not defined in <797>. It is up to you to determine the appropriate work-space requirements.

11.8 SEGREGATED COMPOUNDING AREAS FOR NONHAZARDOUS CSPs

11.8-1 What are the minimum room requirements for an SCA?

An SCA is a type of secondary engineering control but does not have all the controls of a cleanroom suite. It needs to be an area that is dedicated to sterile compounding. A separate room is recommended but not required. A visible perimeter must be defined to establish the boundary of the SCA. It cannot have unsealed windows, doors that open to the outside, or located next to areas that could compromise the environmental control. (Areas like warehouses, restrooms, or dietary service areas could cause contamination—either particles, microbial, or both—to flow into the SCA.)

11.8-2 What can be mixed in an SCA?

Nonhazardous CSPs can be mixed in an SCA. If your Assessment of Risk allows the entity-exemption of NIOSH HDs that are not Table 1 antineoplastics,[19] they can be mixed in an SCA as long as you have defined the alternative containment and/or work practices required.

11.8-3 Can all CSPs be mixed in an SCA?

No. NIOSH Table 1 antineoplastics[19] and other drugs your Assessment of Risk does not entity-exempt cannot be mixed in an SCA but can be mixed in a C-SCA.

11.8-4 What does a cleanroom suite have that an SCA doesn't have?

A cleanroom suite, in addition to air changes, pressure requirements, and other controls, has an anteroom and buffer room, HEPA-filtered ceiling air, and is ISO classified.

11.8-5 What is the purpose of a perimeter around the hood?

The visible perimeter defines the boundaries of the SCA, which must be restricted to activities related to sterile compounding.

11.8-6 Where does the sink need to be placed in an SCA?

The sink cannot be within the perimeter around the hood in an SCA. It needs to be accessible but no closer than 1 meter to the PEC.

11.8-7 Are there separate requirements for an SCA used for chemo?

An SCA cannot be used for mixing NIOSH Table 1 antineoplastic CSPs.[19] Those must be mixed in a negative pressure buffer room of a cleanroom suite or in a C-SCA.

11.8-8 What is the ISO requirement for an SCA?

An SCA is not required to be ISO classified.

11.9 CONTAINMENT SEGREGATED COMPOUNDING AREAS FOR HAZARDOUS CSPs

11.9-1 What are the minimum room requirements for a C-SCA?

<800> defines the requirements for mixing hazardous drugs.[4] A C-SCA used for compounding hazardous drugs must have four minimum criteria:

▸ Room with fixed walls that is separate from nonhazardous compounding

▸ Negative pressure between 0.010″ to 0.030″ wc negative to adjacent space

▸ Vented to the outside

▸ At least 12 ACPH (30 ACPH is required for a negative pressure buffer room in a cleanroom suite.)

11.9-2 Can I use a C-SCA for mixing all CSPs—both hazardous and not?

Once drugs and supplies are exposed to the environment used for storage and compounding HDs, they would all need to be considered potentially contaminated with HD residue. You can have two areas: an SCA for nonhazardous drugs and a C-SCA for HDs.

11.9-3 What does a cleanroom suite have that a C-SCA doesn't have?

A cleanroom suite, in addition to other controls, has an anteroom and buffer room, HEPA-filtered ceiling air, and is ISO classified.

11.9-4 Where does the sink need to be placed in a C-SCA?

The sink needs to be directly outside or inside the C-SCA but no closer than 1 meter to the C-PEC or entrance to any negative room.

11.9-5 What is the ISO requirement for a C-SCA?

An SCA is not required to be ISO classified.

11.10 PASS-THROUGH CHAMBERS

11.10-1 What is a pass-through?

It is a chamber—usually around 2 feet by 2 feet by 2 feet in size—that is placed between two rooms to allow supplies to be passed into an area and completed CSPs to be passed out.

11.10-2 What components make a pass-through cleanroom-compliant?

It needs to have sealed doors on both sides that aren't open at the same time. Interlocked doors are best, which prohibit both sides from being opened at the same time. It needs to be cleanable; stainless steel is best. A window allows you to see what's inside the chamber.

11.10-3 How big can a pass-through chamber be?

There is no restriction in <797>, but use of a chamber (about 2 feet by 2 feet in size) minimizes the potential environmental challenges.

11.10-4 Can a pass-through go from unclassified space into a cleanroom?

Yes, but be sure to place it to minimize potential issues with contamination. HEPA-filtered pass-throughs are available and could be considered. The FDA document on insanitary conditions[34] should be consulted for additional information.

11.10-5 What testing is needed for a pass-through chamber?

Your certifier needs to include the pass-through testing in your initial and every 6-month certification to be sure the use of the pass-through under dynamic conditions does not compromise the air handling in the room. If you have a HEPA filtered pass-through, your certifier needs to confirm that the HEPA filters meet the manufacturer's requirements and document that using CETA[32] or equivalent criteria. Include surfaces in the pass-through in your environmental monitoring.

11.10-6 How can I tell if the pass-through is contributing to problems in the IV room?

Check several things:

▶ Is your staff following the policies you established to ensure appropriate use of the pass-through?

▶ Does your certification report show that the pass-through was included as part of your certification?

▶ Does your environmental monitoring show any microbial growth?

11.10-7 We have a window that slides open between the anteroom and buffer room. Is this a pass-through chamber?

No. It is unacceptable to use. Have it replaced with a solid wall or a cleanroom-compliant pass-through chamber.

11.10-8 Is a window OK in the pass-through chamber?

Yes, as long as it is cleanable and an integral part of the pass-through chamber. You want a window in each side; otherwise, you would not know if there was anything inside the chamber.

11.10-9 Does the pass-through chamber need to be HEPA-filtered?

It is not required by <797> but may be required by your state. Consider use of a HEPA-filtered pass-through if it enters into a negative area. Consult the FDA document on insanitary conditions[34] for additional information.

11.10-10 I have a HEPA-filtered pass-through. Can I turn off the HEPA filter when it's not in use?

Check the manufacturer's information and confirm the use with your certifier.

11.10-11 Do HEPA-filtered pass-throughs need to be ISO classified?

Yes. That's the point of having a HEPA-filtered pass-through.

11.10-12 How big are pass-through chambers?

Generally, they are about 2 feet by 2 feet by 2 feet in size.

11.10-13 Is it OK to pass supplies through a pass-through?

Yes. That's the point of a pass-through. Be sure your policies define how you want it used.

11.10-14 Our pass-through isn't interlocked, but we only allow opening one side at a time. Is this OK?

An interlocked chamber is not required by <797>, but it is the best way to ensure proper use. If you don't have a device that is interlocked, your policies must define the specific requirements and you need to ensure your staff is using it correctly.

11.10-15 We have a pass-through that is interlocked, but I can feel air moving in from the other room. Is this OK?

No. There is something wrong. It may be that the chamber is not properly sealed.

11.10-16 Is a cart-sized pass-through OK to have?

Yes, with proper design. <797> does not define the size, but a cart-sized pass-through can compromise the air flow in a cleanroom and is challenging for cleaning. If you use this, your facility needs to be designed to allow proper use.

11.10-17 Is a pass-through refrigerator OK to have?

It is not prohibited in <797> but is prohibited in <800> for use into negative pressure rooms. Consider the risks even in a nonhazardous area because openings the size of the refrigerator doors will likely affect air flow in the room. It needs to be meticulously cleaned and included in environmental monitoring to ensure you are not compromising the environmental control.

11.11 REFRIGERATOR AND FREEZER PLACEMENT

11.11-1 Is it OK to have refrigerators or freezers in a sterile compounding area?

Yes, and their placement must be considered when designing or renovating the area. A wall air return needs to be placed near the spot where the compressor could contribute particles into the room. There are refrigerators on the market that have a solid-state design and don't have compressors. You might want to consider them because they don't contribute particles to the room. A refrigerator is required by <800> for storage of NIOSH Table 1 antineoplastics[19] in your negative pressure buffer room, C-SCA, or in a separate HD storage room.

11.11-2 What type of refrigerator is required?

The refrigerator should be medical grade. Consider use of a refrigerator that uses a solid-state design (without a compressor) because those do not contribute particles to the room.

11.11-3 What does a "low wall return" for a refrigerator mean?

The air return is low on the wall to capture particles generated by the refrigerator.

11.11-4 Is a pass-through refrigerator OK to have?

It is not prohibited in <797> but is prohibited in <800> for use into negative pressure rooms. Consider the risks even in a nonhazardous area because the size of the refrigerator doors will likely affect air flow in the room. It needs to be meticulously cleaned and included in environmental monitoring to ensure you are not compromising the environmental control.

11.12 OTHER COMPOUNDING AREA EQUIPMENT

11.12-1 What other kind of equipment is used for sterile compounding?

Equipment other than hoods includes repeater pumps, automated compounding devices, mixers, and many other devices depending on the scope of compounding. Some state regulations list specific articles that must be maintained.

11.12-2 How do I know that mechanical equipment is OK to use?

When equipment is received, be sure to follow the manufacturer's instructions for set-up, have biomechanical engineering (or a department with a similar function) ensure the correct operation, provide in-services to staff, and document competence of staff to properly operate the equipment.

11.12-3 How can I be sure the equipment is USP-compliant?

USP does not certify equipment; that needs to be done by your independent certifier.

11.12-4 Can I have a telephone in the sterile compounding area?

There is no restriction in <797> concerning the equipment you may have in your sterile compounding room. The key is that the room meets the certification criteria under dynamic condition. However, consider use of a hands-free intercom rather than a standard telephone. For medication safety reasons, some organizations only allow outgoing calls from the sterile compounding area because incoming calls could interrupt compounding.

11.12-5 Can I have a printer in the sterile compounding area?

There is no restriction in <797> concerning the equipment you may have in your sterile compounding room. The key is that the room meets the certification criteria under dynamic conditions. However, review your processes to be sure you only have the minimum additional equipment needed.

11.12-6 We use a system that has a computer tablet in the hood. Is this OK?

There is no restriction in <797> concerning the equipment you may have in your sterile compounding hood or room. The key is that the room meets the certification criteria under dynamic condition. Because the equipment is in your PEC, include it in your environmental monitoring to be sure it isn't adversely impacting the state of control of the PEC.

11.12-7 Is it OK to have a warmer in the sterile compounding area?

Is it necessary for sterile compounding? Evaluate the need. If it must be inside the sterile compounding area, be sure it is not adversely impacting the state of control of your room.

11.12-8 Is it OK to have an incubator in the sterile compounding area?

No. You don't want anything in the room that contains growth media. If you have an incubator in the pharmacy, move it to an area outside the sterile compounding space.

11.12-9 Is there a requirement to calibrate the equipment?

Thermometers, humidity devices, pressure gauges, and any other monitoring equipment need to be calibrated or verified at least every 12 months or more frequently if recommended by the manufacturer of the equipment, any regulatory agency, your accreditation organization, or organizational policy. Your certifier needs to supply you with documentation of the equipment used during certification; this should be a part of your every 6-month report.

11.13 COMPOUNDING IMMEDIATE-USE CSPs IN AMBIENT AIR

11.13-1 What does *ambient air* mean?

Ambient air is a condition that doesn't meet the ISO classification and other requirements of PECs or SECs; for example, the area in a nursing unit or procedural area where immediate-use CSPs are prepared.

11.13-2 Why is it OK to mix CSPs outside of an IV room?

In critical care areas or procedural areas, there is a need to mix sterile products for urgent patient use. <797> allows for this and for preparation per approved labeling of sterile preparations to adequately take care of patients. However, use of immediate-use preparation should not be used when appropriate facilities and personnel are available to mix the CSPs under the proper controlled conditions.

11.13-3 Is the OR considered ambient air?

Yes. The operating room (OR) is ambient air so limited to immediate use and preparation per approved labeling.

11.13-4 What minimum requirements should an area used for immediate-use preparations have?

The area needs to be clean, uncluttered, and functionally separate.

11.13-5 If IVs are mixed in ambient air, do those areas need to be included in environmental monitoring?

<797> does not require this. If used for trending, recognize that you will likely have growth because the room is not ISO-classified.

11.13-6 Is a doctor's office considered ambient air?

Yes. Except for the preparation of allergenic extracts, any clinic area without a PEC and SEC is ambient air and limited to immediate use and preparation per approved labeling.

11.14 ALLERGENIC EXTRACTS COMPOUNDING AREA

11.14-1 Do allergen extracts have to be prepared in an IV room?

Ideally, allergen extracts will be prepared in a PEC within a cleanroom suite or SCA dedicated only to that type of preparation. However, because of the type of CSP (self-preserved) and need for patient care purposes (a longer BUD to allow for appropriate patient treatment), a special type of control is permitted. <797> defines the allergenic extracts compounding area (AECA).[3]

11.14-2 Do allergen extracts have to be prepared in an SCA?

Ideally, allergen extracts should be prepared in a PEC within a cleanroom suite or SCA dedicated only to that type of preparation. However, because of the type of CSP (preserved) and need for patient care purposes (a longer BUD to allow for appropriate patient treatment), a special type of control is permitted: an AECA.[3]

11.14-3 The allergists at our health system want to comply with <797>. What choices do they have for facility design?

There are four choices:

1. A cleanroom suite dedicated to preparation of allergen extracts
2. An SCA dedicated to the preparation of allergen extracts
3. Use of a PEC
4. Use of an AECA

11.14-4 What is an AECA?

An AECA is a dedicated area, used to compound allergen extracts prescription sets that is similar to the facility design for an SCA. A separate room is recommended but not required. A visible perimeter must be defined to establish the boundary of the AECA. It cannot have unsealed windows, have doors that go to the outside, or be next to areas that could compromise the environmental control. (Areas like warehouses, restrooms, or dietary service areas could cause contamination—either particles, microbial, or both—to flow into the AECA.) A sink needs to be accessible for hand hygiene but cannot be closer than 1 meter to the work surface of the AECA.

11.14-5 If a pharmacy prepares allergen extracts, does it need to be done in a regular IV room or is an AECA required?

It should not be done in your regular IV room because you would be introducing mold, pet dander, and other components of allergen extracts prescription sets into your IV room. An AECA is not the only option you have, but it is one option. Consider establishing a separate SCA containing a PEC and use it only for preparation of allergen extracts prescription sets. For the PEC, consider use of a BSC (which does not necessarily have to be externally vented for this purpose).

11.14-6 Does an AECA require a hood?

An AECA is an alternative to a hood.

11.14-7 When is it OK to use an AECA?

The only use of an AECA is for preparation of allergen extracts prescription sets.

11.14-8 Can only doctor's offices have an AECA?

This is not limited to a prescriber's office. It can be used in a hospital, but consider use of a separate SCA with a PEC for more control of the area.

11.15 SEGREGATED RADIOPHARMACEUTICAL PROCESSING AREA

11.15-1 Can radiopharmaceuticals be mixed in the regular pharmacy IV room?

No. Radiopharmaceuticals can only be manipulated in an area defined in the organization's radioactive materials (RAM) license.

11.15-2 Can radiopharmaceuticals be mixed in the laboratory's BSC?

No. Radiopharmaceuticals can only be manipulated in an area defined in the organization's RAM license.

11.15-3 Does the nuclear medicine department need an IV room?

It depends on what they manipulate. Most nuclear medicine departments do not compound CSPs; they manipulate conventionally manufactured products (such as kits for the *in vivo* labeling of red blood cells with technetium Tc-99m) and distribute radiopharmaceuticals prepared by a contracted nuclear pharmacy. If their activities are limited to these functions, they do not necessarily require a PEC, ISO classified area, or a segregated radiopharmaceutical processing area (SRPA). If their activities are more complex than this, they need the appropriate facilities as defined in *USP General Chapter <825> Radiopharmaceuticals—Preparation, Compounding, Dispensing, and Repackaging.* See <825>[5] for full information.

11.15-4 Does the nuclear medicine department need a hood?

It depends on what they manipulate. Most nuclear medicine departments do not compound CSPs; they manipulate conventionally manufactured products (such as kits for the *in vivo* labeling of red blood cells with technetium Tc-99m) and distribute radiopharmaceuticals prepared by a contracted nuclear pharmacy. If their activities are limited to these functions, they do not necessarily require a PEC, ISO classified area, or an SRPA. If their activities are more complex than this, they need the appropriate facilities as defined in <825>. See <825>[5] for full information.

11.15-5 What is an SRPA?

An SRPA is a dedicated area limited to sterile radiopharmaceutical preparation, preparation with minor deviations, dispensing, and repackaging that is similar to the facility design for an SCA. A separate room is recommended but not required. A visible perimeter must be defined to establish the boundary of the SRPA. It cannot have unsealed windows, have doors that go to the outside, or be next to areas that could compromise the environmental control. (Areas like warehouses, restrooms, or dietary service areas could cause contamination—either particles, microbial, or both—to flow into the SRPA.) A sink needs to be accessible for hand hygiene but cannot be closer than 1 meter to the work surface of the SRPA. See <825>[5] for full information.

11.15-6 Does my nuclear medicine department require an SRPA?

It depends on what they manipulate. Most nuclear medicine departments do not compound CSPs; they manipulate conventionally manufactured products (such as kits for the *in vivo* labeling) and distribute radiopharmaceuticals prepared by a contracted nuclear pharmacy. If their activities are limited to these functions, they do not necessarily require a PEC, ISO classified area, or an SRPA. If their activities are more complex than this, they need the appropriate facilities as defined in <825>. See <825>[5] for full information.

DAILY NONVIABLE MONITORING *12*

12.1   What monitoring is required to be done daily?

You need to be sure your sterile compounding area is always in a state of control identified by <797>, best practices, and your policies and procedures.

Minimum items that need to be documented at least daily include the following:

▶ Temperature in storage areas for sterile products below the maximum permitted in manufacturer's labeling, which is generally less than 25°C

▶ Temperature in the sterile compounding areas, which should be less than 20°C

▶ Proper temperature in refrigerators (between 2°C and 8°C), freezers (generally between –25°C and –10°C, but some drugs require different temperature), warmers (based on the drugs stored), and incubators (varies based on the requirement of the media)

▶ Relative humidity in the sterile compounding areas, which should be less than 60%

▶ Calibration of sterile compounding equipment (e.g., automated compounders, repeater pumps)

▶ Pressure differential

   ▲ Anteroom needs to be at least 0.020″ water column (wc) greater than the adjacent room.

   ▲ Positive pressure buffer room needs to be at least 0.020″ wc greater than the anteroom.

   ▲ Negative pressure buffer room needs to be between 0.010″ and 0.030″ wc less than the anteroom.

   ▲ C-SCA needs to be between 0.010″ and 0.030″ wc less than the adjacent room

   ▲ Negative pressure storage rooms must be at least 0.010″ wc negative to the surrounding nonhazardous rooms.

   ▲ Other facility or equipment monitoring as required by manufacturer's recommendations, regulatory agencies, accreditation organizations, or your policies and procedures.

12.2   What's the difference between nonviable and viable monitoring?

Nonviable monitoring are other parameters such as temperature, humidity, pressure, and equipment elements. *Viable* monitoring is the environmental monitoring for microbial contamination.

DOI 10.37573/9781585287260.012

12.3 What's the difference between certification and monitoring?

Certification is the process conducted at least every 6 months by a qualified individual who examines the primary engineering controls (PECs) and secondary engineering controls (SECs) to be sure they are within the proper specification. Certification is part of *monitoring*, but your monitoring program needs to include other viable and nonviable elements required by <797> and <800>.

12.4 What monitoring is the certifier required to do?

Certification includes the following:

▶ Airflow testing of your PEC and SEC
▶ HEPA filter integrity testing of your PEC and SEC
▶ Total particle count testing of your PEC and SEC
▶ Dynamic air flow testing of your PEC

They should use the CETA[32] Certification Application Guide 003 for Sterile Compounding Facilities or a comparable document.

12.5 Our certifier also does the viable testing. Is this OK?

Yes, but viable testing is different from certification. See Chapter 18 concerning environmental monitoring (EM). EM can be done by you or by your certifier.

12.6 What should the temperature of the sterile compounding areas be?

It should be less than 20°C.

12.7 What do I need to do if it's too cold in the sterile compounding area?

Talk to your facilities personnel who need to adjust the temperature. There is no minimum temperature requirement in <797>.

12.8 What do I need to do if it's too warm in the sterile compounding area?

Define this in your policies and procedures. Consider rechecking the temperature in 1 hour. If it is still out of range, notify your facilities personnel concerning the excursion. Prolonged temperature above 20°C contributes a risk of microbial proliferation.

12.9 Do I need to monitor the temperature of storage areas outside the intravenous (IV) room?

Yes. This is a general pharmacy issue. The medications and supplies must be stored within the temperature range defined by the supplier. Most drugs cannot be stored above 25°C. Brief excursions are allowed. See *USP General Chapter <659> Packaging and Storage Requirements.*[35]

12.10 What should the humidity be in the sterile compounding area?

It should be under 60% relative humidity.

12.11 What should I do if the humidity is too low?

There is no minimum relative humidity requirement in <797>. The concern with sterile preparations is too *high* a humidity because it can contribute to microbial proliferation. A low humidity may be a personnel comfort issue but it is not a risk to the CSPs.

12.12 My facilities department says the humidity has to be at least 20%. They want to add a humidifier. Is that OK?

No. You cannot add in water sources to the sterile compounding area. There are other departments in the health system where low humidity is a risk (such as a potential for fires in the surgical suite). Low humidity may be a personnel comfort issue but it is not a risk to the CSPs.

12.13 What should I do if the humidity is too high?

It needs to be corrected. Relative humidity above 60% can contribute to microbial proliferation.

12.14 Can we use a dehumidifier to correct humidity that is too high?

No. A free-standing dehumidifier cannot be used. The correction must be made in the air handling system.

12.15 What should I do if the pressure in my anteroom or positive pressure buffer room is too positive?

Talk with your certifier for the best answer. Often, the certifier, your facilities department, and an air balancer work together to adjust the pressure. Having too high a positive pressure is not a violation of <797> because it requires only a minimum positive pressure of 0.020″ wc to adjacent rooms.

12.16 What should I do if the pressure in my negative pressure buffer room or C-SCA is too negative?

Talk with your certifier for the best answer. Often, the certifier, your facilities department, and an air balancer work together to adjust the pressure. This is a serious issue because negative pressure greater than 0.030″ wc presents a risk of pulling contaminants into the negative room from adjacent areas (including ceilings). Other manifestations often include bacterial or fungal growth from those adjacent areas and difficulty in closing or opening doors. A pressure range between 0.010″ and 0.030″ wc negative to adjacent rooms is required by <800>.[4]

12.17 If temperature, humidity, or pressure is out of range, do I have to report this to someone?

Your state may require it. Your organizational policy may require it. In any case, be sure to document the values and correction.

12.18 How often does our automated compounding device (ACD) need to be tested?

The ACD needs to be checked and documented daily (when used) to be sure it is working properly. For preventive maintenance, follow the manufacturer's recommendations and include the device in your biomechanical engineering's (or similar department) roster of patient-related equipment.

12.19 How often does our repeater pump need to be tested?

The repeater pump needs to be checked and documented daily (when used) to be sure it is working properly. For preventive maintenance, follow the manufacturer's recommendations and include the device in your biomechanical engineering's (or similar department) roster of patient-related equipment.

CERTIFICATION OF ENGINEERING CONTROLS *13*

13.1 What does *certification* mean? How is it different from the monitoring I have to do every day?

Certification is the process conducted by a qualified technician who evaluates the primary engineering controls (PECs) and secondary engineering controls (SECs) for compliance with key elements required by <797>.

13.2 What qualifications does a certifier need?

Many companies provide certification services. All should use the criteria included in the CETA Certification Application Guides (CAGs)[32] or equivalent documents including airflow testing of the PEC and SEC, high efficiency particulate air (HEPA)-filter integrity testing of the PEC and SEC, total particle count testing of the PEC and SEC, and dynamic airflow smoke pattern testing of the PEC.[36]

CETA has a board certification for certifiers who have completed didactic and practical testing concerning all aspects of sterile compounding facility requirements. The designation CNBT (CETA National Board of Testing) indicates that the certifier has successfully completed all the requirements of this distinction.

13.3 What is CETA?

CETA is the Controlled Environment Testing Association, which is the professional organization for the sterile compounding certification industry.

13.4 What are CETA CAGs?

CETA does not set standards; they use existing standards, such as <797> and <800>, and develop guidance documents that incorporate all of the required elements. CAGs are their certification guides, which include those for evaluating the different types of PECs and sterile compounding facilities.

13.5 What should my certification report include?

Your report should include all the elements in the applicable CETA CAGs that apply to your devices and facility, confirmation that it was done under dynamic operating conditions, and that calibrated equipment was used for the test. The certifier should indicate which devices and areas pass all requirements, which may need attention for future certification evaluations, and which fail to meet the requirements. If your certifier does not provide a summary sheet, consider completing the information in Exhibit 13-1.

DOI 10.37573/9781585287260.013

EXHIBIT 13-1. Summary of IV Hood/Room Certification

SUMMARY OF IV HOOD/ROOM CERTIFICATION

Location:

Date of Certification:	Certifier:

PEC	Brand	Test Standard		Meets ISO 5
LAFW		CETA CAG 003 or equivalent		
CAI		CETA CAG 002 or equivalent		
BSC A2		NSF 49		
BSC B2		NSF 49		
CACI		CETA CAG 002 or equivalent		

SEC	Test	Requirement	Result	Pass/Fail
Anteroom	HEPA Leak Test	Less than 0.1%		
	Air Changes	30 ACPH		
	Pressure to adjacent area	At least 0.020" positive		
	ISO Class	ISO 8 if only positive buffer room/s ISO 7 if enters into any negative space		
Positive Buffer	HEPA Leak Test	Less than 0.1%		
	Air Changes	30 ACPH		
	Source of air changes	At least 15 from air handling system Up to 15 may come from PEC		
	Pressure to anteroom	At least 0.020" positive		
	ISO Class	ISO 7		
Negative Buffer	HEPA Leak Test	Less than 0.1%		
	Air Changes	30 ACPH		
	Pressure to anteroom	Between 0.010-0.030" negative		
	ISO Class	ISO 7		
SCA				
C-SCA	Air Changes	12 ACPH		
	Pressure to adjacent area	Between 0.010-0.030" negative		
HD Storage	Pressure to adjacent area	At least 0.010" negative		

13.6   What does *dynamic conditions* mean?

Similar situations as occur during your normal operating conditions. For example, if three people are usually in the buffer room, three people need to be in the room during certification. If an ACD or a repeater pump is kept in your PEC, that pump needs to be in the PEC during the testing.

13.7   Can I compound while the certifier is working in the room?

No, but you can simulate compounding or perform other activities (such as transfer of materials) that would normally occur.

13.8   Does the certifier need access to the ceiling above the intravenous (IV) room?

They need some way to access the ceiling HEPA filters. That may mean removing some panels in the ceiling. Ideally, have ports installed to allow the certifier to test the integrity of the filters without the need to physically access the space above the ceiling.

13.9   Is there a way to test the ceiling HEPA filters without crawling in the ceiling?

You can add ports that allow the certifier to test the integrity of the filters without the need to physically access the space above the ceiling.

13.10   My hood failed certification. Can I use it?

No, not until it is fixed and recertified. If a PEC fails certification, it means that one or more of the key required elements were not met. Correct the deficiency and have the hood recertified.

13.11   My room failed certification. Can I use it?

Maybe. If the room failed certification but the PEC passed certification, you may be able to consider the area as a segregated compounding area until you are able to have the room fixed and recertified. However, evaluate the reason the room failed to make a decision that supports safe practices.

13.12   We use an ACD. Should we take it out of the hood when the certifier tests the hood?

No. It needs to be kept in the PEC during certification because that is your normal operating condition.

13.13   We use a repeater pump. Should we take it out of the hood when the certifier tests the hood?

No. It needs to be kept in the PEC during certification because that is your normal operating condition.

13.14 We use an IV software system that has equipment in the hood. Should we take it out of the hood when the certifier tests the hood?

No. It needs to be kept in the PEC during certification because that is your normal operating condition.

13.15 Should the certifier do our environmental monitoring?

They can, but that is a different process than certification. See Chapter 18.

13.16 If the power goes off in our hood or room, does it need to be recertified before we can use it again?

It depends on the specific situation. This is not addressed in <797> so detail this in your policies and procedures. If the power is off for a short period of time (e.g., 1 hour or less), perform a total cleaning of the PEC prior to resuming sterile compounding. If the power is off for an extended period of time (e.g., a weather situation that lasts several days), that could present significant risk of microbial proliferation. In that case, consider a total cleaning of the PEC and SEC and take environmental samples. Based on your policy—and in conjunction with your facilities personnel, infection control practitioner, and designated person overseeing sterile compounding—assess the need for recertification prior to resuming sterile compounding.

13.17 Our certifier says our chemo room is "too negative." Is this correct?

If the room is more than 0.030″ wc negative than adjacent space, it does not meet the requirements of <800>.

13.18 Do we have to get our hoods and rooms certified before we use them?

Yes. The certifier needs to certify the PECs and SECs prior to use. You will see the term *commissioning* used which indicates an evaluation of the devices and facilities prior to first use.

13.19 When does a hood need to be certified?

It needs to be certified on commissioning (prior to first use), at least every 6 months, and whenever it is moved or serviced.

13.20 When does a room need to be certified?

It needs to be certified on commissioning (prior to first use), at least every 6 months, and whenever the configuration of the room is changed that could affect airflow or other quality issues.

13.21 Can my facilities department check my hood?

Unlikely, because you need an independent qualified certifier who uses the criteria in the CETA CAGs or equivalent document.

13.22 We have a powder hood in our negative pressure storage room. Does it need to be retested every 6 months or every year?

If this is used only for nonsterile compounding, <795> applies.[2] PECs used only for nonsterile compounding must be certified at least every 12 months. However, because your certifier will certify your PECs for sterile compounding every 6 months, consider including the PEC for nonsterile use every 6-month frequency as well. If this is used for presterilization activities for CSPs, the room needs to be at least ISO 8 and the powder containment hood would need to be certified every 6 months.

COMPOUNDING 14

14.1 GENERAL INFORMATION

14.1-1 How many people are allowed in the sterile compounding area?

That depends on your devices and facility. Anyone entering the sterile compounding area needs to be authorized to be in the area. Your policies and procedures need to define the routine and maximum number of personnel in each area. That information needs to be available to your certifier so he or she knows the number of personnel who need to be in the room during certification to identify the dynamic operating conditions.

14.1-2 Can students compound sterile preparations? If not, how can they learn?

Any personnel—employees or students—need to successfully complete training including hand hygiene and garbing, post-garbing gloved fingertip and thumb testing, and aseptic processing (media fill, gloved fingertip and thumb testing, surface sampling) prior to independently compounding for patients. Some learning can be completed by observation and working with simulated conditions.

14.1-3 Are cellphones allowed in the sterile compounding areas?

No. Unnecessary items should not be allowed in the sterile compounding area. You need to define this in your policies and procedures. Consider the reason for needing a cell phone. It certainly would not be for making personal calls while compounding, so is it really needed?

14.1-4 Is it OK to play music in the sterile compounding area?

It is not recommended. Think of the medication safety issues—it could be a distraction.

14.1-5 Is mixing immediate-use compounded sterile preparations (CSPs) considered compounding?

It is compounding but some of the requirements (such as media fill, gloved fingertip and thumb test, and surface sample) are not required. It does not need to be done in a PEC or within a compounding suite or segregated compounding area. The area for immediate-use preparation needs to be clean, uncluttered, and functionally separate from other activities.

DOI 10.37573/9781585287260.014

14.1-6 What special policies and procedures are needed for compounding intrathecal or epidural CSPs?

<797> does not distinguish among different sterile dosage forms. You need to address this in your policies and procedures.

14.1-7 Are vial tops sterile when they come from the manufacturer?

No. They are only dust covers. The septum of any vial needs to be appropriately disinfected prior to use.

14.1-8 Are there some drugs that I should not compound?

Yes. The Food and Drug Administration (FDA) has details on what can and cannot be compounded. There are different requirements for 503A compounding pharmacies and 503B outsourcing facilities concerning use of bulk substances.[37] State-licensed physicians and pharmacists who compound under section 503A of the Federal Food, Drug, and Cosmetic Act (FD&C Act) may only compound drug products using bulk drug substances that

▶ Comply with an applicable *United States Pharmacopeia (USP)* or *National Formulary (NF)* monograph if one exists

▶ Comply with <797> and <800>

▶ Are components of FDA-approved drug products if an applicable *USP* or *NF* monograph does not exist

▶ Appear on the FDA's list of bulk drug substances, which can be used in compounding (the 503A list[38]) if such a monograph does not exist and the substance is not a component of an FDA-approved drug product

In addition, bulk drug substances must be accompanied by a valid Certificate of Analysis (CoA) and must have been manufactured by an establishment registered with FDA under section 510 of the FD&C Act.

A pharmacist must not compound any commercially available product or any preparations that contain drug products on the FDA's *List of Drug Products That Have Been Withdrawn or Removed from the Market for Reasons of Safety or Effectiveness,* codified in Title 21 Code of Federal Regulations (CFR) 216.24.[39] However, a pharmacist may compound a commercially available product if, in the professional judgment of the prescriber, the product is modified to produce a significant difference between the compounded product for the patient and the comparable commercially available product.

14.1-9 Is the bulk list the same for pharmacies and for outsourcing facilities?

There are two separate lists: one for 503A pharmacies and one for 503B outsourcing facilities. 503B outsourcing facilities can only use bulk drug substances for agents that are in shortage or that appear on a list developed by the FDA for bulk drug substances for which there is a clinical need.

14.1-10 Is prepackaging medications into syringe containers considered compounding?

Yes. See *USP General Chapter <1178> Good Repackaging Practices*[40] and the FDA guidance documents concerning repackaging.[8]

14.1-11 Does ASHP have guidelines dealing with sterile compounding?

Yes. See the *ASHP Guidelines on Compounding Sterile Preparations*[41] and *Guidelines on Handling Hazardous Drugs.*[42] Some of the documents predate <797> so the USP standard needs to be followed when it is more stringent than the information in the ASHP document.

14.1-12 Are premixed solutions that I can buy from manufacturers considered compounded?

No. Items from a manufacturer are *products*, not compounded preparations.

14.1-13 Are premixed solutions that I can buy from an outsourcing facility considered compounded?

Yes. They are compounds. However, these items from 503B outsourcing facilities are called *products* (not preparations) in some FDA documents.

14.1-14 Is reconstituting a system like an ADD-Vantage™, MINI-BAG Plus, VIAL-MATE, or addEASE® considered compounding?

No, as long as you are attaching and activating these proprietary bag and vial systems for immediate administration. If you are docking the systems for future activation and administration, it is considered compounding but you can use the beyond-use dates (BUDs) established by the manufacturer.

14.1-15 If I crush tablets or open capsules to make a CSP, is that an active pharmaceutical ingredient (API)?

No. Crushing, splitting, opening, or otherwise manipulating an FDA-approved drug does not create an API, the raw chemical that is used to produce the FDA-approved drug.

14.1-16 Is there an algorithm I can use to determine if it's appropriate to compound?

Consider this:

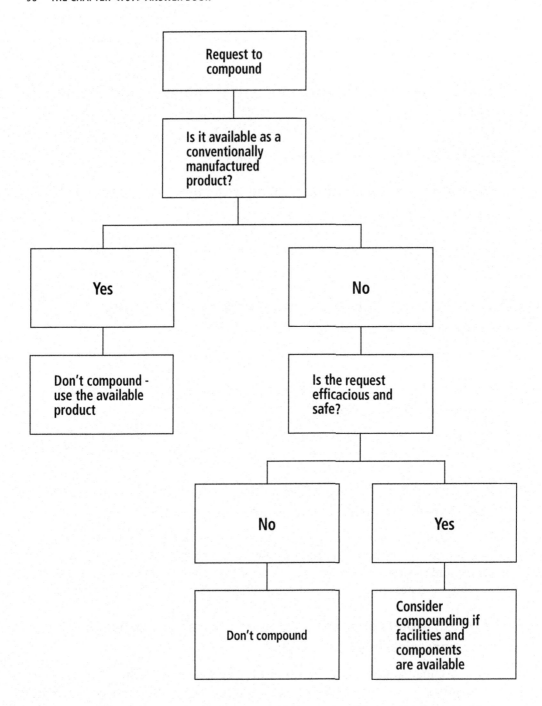

14.2 NONSTERILE-TO-STERILE COMPOUNDING

14.2-1 How do I know if an ingredient is nonsterile?

Sterile components are those conventionally manufactured products that are intended for parenteral use. They are marked as sterile on the final container. Anything else is not sterile. This includes APIs from suppliers, drugs not intended for parenteral use, and containers and closures that are not sterile.

14.2-2 Do I need a Certificate of Analysis for every ingredient in a compound?

All APIs used must have a lot-specific Certificate of Analysis (CoA). FDA-approved drugs do not need a CoA. Ingredients other than APIs or FDA-approved drugs should have a CoA.

14.2-3 How are CSPs that start with nonsterile components sterilized?

Ideally, they are terminally sterilized using steam (an autoclave), dry heat (an oven), or irradiation. If terminal sterilization cannot be done, they can be filtered. Note that filtration is *not* considered terminal sterilization.

14.2-4 What is the difference between terminal sterilization and filtration?

Terminal sterilization achieves a low probability of a nonsterile unit (PNSU). *Filtered* items that do not have the same assurance for this.

14.2-5 What is a bubble point test?

The bubble point test is a test of the filter that has been used to prepare a nonsterile-to-sterile CSP. You need to test every filter used for sterile compounding to be sure the integrity of the filter was not compromised during compounding.

14.2-6 Do containers need to be sterile?

Yes. All components of a CSP need to be sterile and pyrogen-free, including the containers and closures.

14.2-7 Is it OK to use an amber dropper bottle for sterile CSPs?

A standard dropper bottle is *not* sterile. You can obtain appropriate sterile containers and closures from several pharmacy suppliers.

14.2-8 If I batch 50 cefazolin syringes, do I need to do sterility tests?

If you are preparing a batch of CSPs under Category 2 conditions and assigning a beyond-use date that does not exceed the maximum BUD listed in <797> and all the components are stable for that length of time, you do not necessarily need to perform sterility testing. (See Chapter 15.)

14.2-9 Are there additional requirements when working with blood components?

Blood components include platelet, red cells, white cells, autologous serum, etc. This is different from a commercially available blood product like albumin or intravenous immunoglobulin (IVIG). If you are compounding with blood components, you need to separate those activities from other compounding activities and develop and implement specific policies and procedures to avoid cross-contamination. See the Centers for Disease Control and Prevention (CDC) Biosafety in Microbiological and Biomedical Laboratories (BMBL) document[43] for additional information.

14.2-10 Are there additional requirements when working with albumin, IVIG, vaccines, or other biologics?

Compounding with biologics introduces additional risk into sterile compounding. For these commercially manufactured products, use the manufacture's information, which likely includes most shorter BUDs than conventionally manufactured products.

14.2-11 Are there additional requirements when working with radio-pharmaceuticals like UltraTag™?

Yes. This cannot be done in your health system's pharmacy IV room. See *USP General Chapter <825> Radiopharmaceuticals—Preparation, Compounding, Dispensing, and Repackaging.*[5]

14.3 MASTER FORMULATION RECORDS

14.3-1 What is a master formulation record?

A master formulation record (MFR) is the recipe for a CSP. It allows a CSP to be reproduced with the same formula on repeated occasions.

14.3-2 When is an MFR needed?

A MFR should be established for CSPs mixed for more than one patient and for all CSPs mixed with any nonsterile ingredient.

14.3-3 What needs to be recorded in an MFR?

Include:

▸ Name, identify, strength or activity, amounts, and dosage forms of all ingredients

▸ Type and size of the container-closure systems

▸ Complete instructions for preparing the CSP, including equipment, supplies, a description of the compounding steps, and any special precautions

- Physical description of the final CSP
- BUD and storage requirements
- Reference source to support the stability of the CSP
- Quality control procedures, such as pH testing and filter integrity testing
- Other information needed to describe the compounding process and ensure repeatability (e.g., adjusting pH and tonicity, sterilization method).

14.3-4 Is there a template form I can use to create an MFR?

See **Exhibit 14-1**.

14.3-5 We have a file with recipes for compounds. Is this the same as an MFR?

Yes, but be sure you have all the elements listed as required by <797>. An update of the recipes will probably be needed.

14.3-6 What references for compounding formulas are available?

USP has over 250 compounding monographs. Some of these are sterile compounds. They are available in the *USP Compounding Compendium*.[1] The *International Journal of Pharmaceutical Compounding*[44] prints formulas in each edition of the journal. Other peer-reviewed sources can also be used.

14.3-7 If I make two different strengths of a CSP, do I need one or two MFRs?

Two. You need a distinct MFR for each unique compound.

14.3-8 Do I need to make an MFR for a one-time order or prescription?

A MFR is required for all CSPs prepared from nonsterile ingredients and for CSPs prepared for more than 1 patient. Your state may have additional requirements.

14.3-9 Can I combine the MFR with a compounding record?

Yes. The MFR and the compounding record (CR) can either be separate or combined documents.

14.3-10 Is it OK to double or halve the listing on the MFR?

It depends if it changes any of the other elements. Your CR needs to note the quantity compounded.

14.3-11 Do the MFRs have to be printed out?

They have to be retrievable. They can be printed or electronic.

14.3-12 What happens if a change has to be made in an MFR?

Then it's a unique compound, so would require a separate MFR.

14.3-13 When changes are necessary, who can make them?

The designated person needs to be responsible for changes in an MFR.

14.3-14 Do I need an MFR for every antibiotic CSP I make?

If you will make it for more than one patient or if it includes any nonsterile component, you should establish a MFR. For example, many hospitals make 10 or more common antibiotic mixtures daily. Establish a separate MFR for each of these.

14.3-15 Does the MFR need to be in a specific format?

No, but it needs to include all the required elements.

14.4 COMPOUNDING RECORDS

14.4-1 What is a compounding record?

A compounding record (CR) is a record of the ingredients used to make a CSP.

14.4-2 When is a CR needed?

A CR is required for all Category 1, 2, and 3 CSPs and for immediate use CSPs prepared for more than one patient.

14.4-3 What needs to be recorded in a CR?

Include:

- Name, strength or activity, and dosage form of the CSP
- Date and time of preparation
- Assigned internal lot number (e.g., prescription, order, or lot number)
- A method to identify the individuals involved in the compounding process and verifying the final CSP
- Name, vendor or manufacturer, lot number, and expiration date of each component for CSPs prepared for more than one patient and for any CSP prepared from nonsterile ingredients
- Weight or volume of each component
- Strength or activity of each component
- Total quantity or number of units compounded
- Assigned BUD and storage requirements

▸ Results of quality control (QC) procedures (e.g., visual inspection, filter integrity testing, pH testing)

If applicable, the CR must also include the following:

▸ Master formulation record reference for the CSP

▸ Calculations made to determine and verify quantities and/or concentrations of components

14.4-4 I've always recorded the information above for batches, but not for "one offs"—a single bag or two for one patient for a specific order. Do I need a CR for those?

You have to have a way to identify the specifics listed. <797> allows you to handle the single order CRs differently than batches, as long as you have a way to trace the information. Detail this in your policies. Some organizations run a duplicate label and maintain it but consider the potential patient safety issues with that process. Some systems create production labels that can be used. Others use camera technology. Your state may also specify maintaining this information for every CSP—including individual IVs—so be sure to follow that if it is more strict than the <797> requirements.

14.4-5 Do I have to record manufacturer's lot numbers for every CSP?

You should record them for all CSPs made for more than one patient or any CSP made from nonsterile ingredients. You have to have a way of identifying the lot number of the component used for other CSPs, and that needs to be detailed in your policies and procedures.

14.4-6 Is there a template form I can use to create a CR?

See **Exhibit 14-2**.

14.4-7 Do the CRs have to be printed out?

They need to be retrievable. They can be printed or electronic.

14.5 ALLERGENIC EXTRACTS

14.5-1 How are allergenic extracts compounded?

The compounding process is no different from those used for other types of CSPs. The difference is the facility design allowed (see Section 11.14) and the BUDs permitted for the prescription sets compounded. See *Compounding Allergenic Extracts* in Section 21 of <797>.[3]

14.6 RADIOPHARMACEUTICALS

14.6-1 How are radiopharmaceuticals compounded?

The compounding process is no different from those used for other types of CSPs. The difference is the personnel protection that must be employed to minimize risk of exposure to radioactivity. See <825>,[5] which details the information concerning facility design, personnel protection, and other details.

14.6-2 Is there a difference between what an outside nuclear pharmacy compounds and what is compounded in the hospital's nuclear medicine department?

That is likely. Very few hospitals have nuclear pharmacists, and those pharmacists generally work in the imaging department. Even fewer hospitals have a separately permitted nuclear pharmacy. Almost all health systems outsource their nuclear pharmacy services to an outside nuclear pharmacy.

The nuclear pharmacies prepare, compound, dispense, and repackage radiopharmaceutical based on Nuclear Regulatory Commission (NRC) requirements, state requirements, USP chapters, and precise policies and procedures. They provide patient-specific doses to your nuclear medicine department. The nuclear pharmacies comply with <825>[5] for radiopharmaceuticals. They may also have an SRPA for other radiopharmaceutials they manipulate.

Your nuclear medicine department likely administers those doses and may manipulate some commercially available products, such as those for the *in vivo* labeling red blood cells with technetium Tc99-m. Based on the complexity of the radiopharmaceutical manipulated, your nuclear medicine department may only need the facilities for immediate-use radiopharmaceuticals. Work with your nuclear medicine department to be sure your health system is in compliance with the appropriate sections of <825>.

EXHIBIT 14-1. Example Master Formulation Record for CSPs

NAME OF PREPARATION (name, strength/activity, dosage form) ☐ USP monograph ☐ Assigned name
INGREDIENTS (name, strength/activity, quantity/amount)
CALCULATIONS ☐ Not applicable
EQUIPMENT
COMPATIBILITY AND STABILITY INFORMATION (including references, if available) ☐ Not applicable
MIXING AND PREPARATION INSTRUCTIONS (Include order and duration of mixing, temperature/other environmental controls, etc.)
CONTAINER AND CLOSURE TYPE (Note both storage and dispensing containers, if different.)
BUD ASSIGNED ☐ 12 hours ☐ 24 hours ☐ 4 days ☐ 10 days ☐ 45 days ☐ BUD assignment based on: _____ ☐ Other reference (list reference and note BUD): _____
PACKAGING/STORAGE REQUIREMENTS ☐ Refrigerate ☐ Freeze ☐ Protect from light
DESCRIPTION OF FINAL PREPARATION
SAMPLE LABEL
QUALITY CONTROL PROCEDURES AND EXPECTED RESULTS

BUD = beyond-use date.

EXHIBIT 14-2. Example Compounding Record for CSPs

PREPARATION (name, strength/activity, dosage form):			Master Formulation Record	
CALCULATIONS:				
INGREDIENT (name, strength/activity, dosage form)	AMOUNT (mL, g, etc.)	MFR	EXP DATE	LOT NUMBER
DATE AND TIME PREPARED:	Affix Label Here			
CONTROL/RX/ORDER NUMBER:				
TOTAL QUANTITY COMPOUNDED:				
PHYSICAL DESCRIPTION:				
BEYOND-USE DATE:				
QUALITY CONTROL RESULTS (if applicable):				
Prepared by:	Checked by:			

EXP = expiration, MFR = manufacturer

BEYOND-USE DATES 15

15.1 GENERAL BEYOND-USE DATE INFORMATION

15.1-1 Is a beyond-use date the same thing as an expiration date?

No. Manufacturers establish expiration dates for their products based on studies of the physical and chemical stability of their products, packaged in the dosage form marketed, when stored based on the requirements of the labeling. The beyond-use dates (BUDs) that compounders assign to preparations are much shorter because the validated testing is not done.

15.1-2 What's the difference among an expiration date, beyond-use date, in-use time, and infusion time?

All of these relate to expiry of products or preparations, but there are differences.

▶ An *expiration date* is set by the manufacturer based on scientific studies at specific storage temperatures.

▶ A *beyond-use date* is set by a compounder. It is shorter than the expiration date because the controls of a manufactured product are not available nor are studies done that support extended dating.

▶ *In-use time* is the time from when a product or preparation is opened or punctured until the point it can no longer be used.

▶ *Infusion time* is the time a product or preparation is being administered to a patient.

15.1-3 What factors go into the determination of a BUD?

Determining a BUD depends on several factors:

▶ Stability of the components—Including drugs, diluents, containers, and closure system

▶ Facility in which the compounded sterile preparation (CSP) is mixed—A cleanroom suite or a segregated compounding area (SCA)

▶ Starting ingredients—All sterile or at least one nonsterile component

▶ Type of preparation—Aseptically prepared (including filtration) or terminally sterilized (autoclaved, use of dry heat over, or irradiation)

▶ Storage temperature—Room temperature, refrigerated, or frozen

▶ Use of a USP monograph

DOI 10.37573/9781585287260.015

15.1-4 We have a cleanroom suite and mix CSPs from commercially available sterile products. What is the maximum BUD we can use?

The BUD always needs to be the shorter of the stability of the CSP components (drugs, diluents, container, and closure system) and the maximum allowable BUD listed in <797>.

In these common scerarios, the maximum BUD depends on the CSP category and the storage temperature.

For Category 1 CSPs (e.g., those mixed in an SCA):

▸ 12 hours or less for CSPs that will be stored at room temperature

▸ 24 hours or less for CSPs that will be stored under refrigeration

For Category 2 CSPs mixed aseptically and containing only sterile starting components and without additional sterility testing:

▸ 4 days or less for CSPs that will be stored at room temperature

▸ 10 days or less for CSPs that will be stored under refrigeration

▸ 45 days or less for CSPs that will be stored frozen

See USP <797> for complete details and other scenarios.

15.1-5 We make all CSPs in an SCA. What is the maximum BUD we can use?

The BUD always needs to be the shorter of the stability of the CSP components (drugs, diluents, container, and closure system) and the maximum allowable BUD listed in <797>. Because an SCA doesn't have all the controls of a cleanroom suite, you are limited to a short beyond-use time of 12 hours or less if stored at room temperature or 24 hours or less if stored under refrigeration.

15.1-6 We make all our chemos in a containment segregated compounding area (C-SCA). What is the maximum BUD we can use?

The BUD always needs to be the shorter of the stability of the CSP components (drugs, diluents, container, and closure system) and the maximum allowable BUD listed in <797>. BUDs are determined by compliance with <797>. Maximum BUDs for CSPs mixed in a C-SCA are the same as those mixed in an SCA of 12 hours or less if stored at room temperature or 24 hours or less if stored under refrigeration.

15.1-7 We have a cleanroom suite and occasionally mix CSPs from nonsterile starting ingredients. What is the maximum BUD we can use?

The BUD always needs to be the shorter of the stability of the CSP components (drugs, diluents, container, and closure system) and the maximum allowable BUD listed in <797>. In this Category 2 scenario, the maximum BUDs in the absence of performing a sterility test depend on the storage temperature, so you will use the following for mixing:

▸ 24 hours or less for CSPs that will be stored at room temperature

▸ 4 days or less for CSPs that will be stored under refrigeration

▸ 45 days or less for CSPs that will be stored frozen

15.1-8 Can we mix CSPs from nonsterile ingredients in an SCA?

Yes, but you are limited to the short BUDs for Category 1 CSPs.

15.1-9 We filter some CSPs mixed from nonsterile ingredients. Is filtration considered terminal sterilization?

No. Filtration is considered aseptic preparation. Terminal sterilization is accomplished by steam, dry heat, or irradiation.

15.1-10 What is a USP monograph?

USP has some sterile compounding monographs available in the *United States Pharmacopeia–National Formulary (USP–NF)* or *USP Compounding Compendium.*[1] They are compounds that have undergone testing and may have BUDs that are longer than those defined in the charts in <797>. To use the BUD, you must make the preparation as directed in the monograph, use the same packaging, and use the same storage temperature.

15.1-11 Where can I find a USP monograph?

They are part of the *USP–NF* and also in the *USP Compounding Compendium,*[1] available at **www.usp.org**.

15.1-12 If we use a USP monograph, can we use the BUD listed in the monograph?

If you mix it with the specified ingredients and follow the monograph exactly (including final testing, if required), you can use the BUD in the USP monograph. Be sure to use the most current version of the monograph.

15.1-13 Can I use a USP monograph and extend the BUD beyond what's listed in the monograph?

No.

15.1-14 Can I use BUDs longer than those listed in <797> if I have peer-reviewed information that states a longer BUD?

If you choose to extend BUDs beyond the limits for Category 2, you must comply with all Category 3 requirements. If you use peer-reviewed information to extend BUDs, you still need to do a stability test in the container and closure system you will use, and need to do sterility tests of every batch. This includes obtaining a stability-indicating method to detect the active ingredients and impurities. See Section 14.4.3 in <797> for complete information.[3]

15.1-15 If a drug's stability information is less than the BUD in <797>, can I still use the <797> BUD?

No. The BUD is *always* the shorter of the stability of the mixture or the allowed BUD times listed in <797>.

15.1-16 What are the required temperature ranges for room temperature, refrigerated, and frozen CSPs?

<659>[35] defines the temperatures:

▶ Controlled room temperature storage is between 20°C and 25°C.

▶ Refrigerated storage is between 2°C and 8°C.

▶ Frozen storage is between –25°C and –10°C.

15.1-17 Are temperatures listed in <797> in Celsius or Fahrenheit?

All temperatures are listed in Celsius.

15.1-18 Does the BUD include the time the drug is infused?

No. The BUDs start when the compounding starts and ends when the CSP starts to be administered to the patient.

15.1-19 How do I know how long a CSP will be infused?

You need to know the rate of infusion so you can appropriately mix the CSP. You need to develop an organizational policy on infusion time (which is often called *hang time*). Resources for information concerning infusion time are available from Centers for Disease Control and Prevention (CDC) in their document *Guidelines for the Prevention of Intravascular Catheter-Related Infections.*[45]

15.1-20 Does the term *used* in <797> include the infusion time?

No. It means the time from compounding up to the point of initiation of administration.

15.1-21 If I make something for one patient from powder and filter it, can I use the terminally sterilized BUD times?

No. You need to use the information for aseptically-prepared BUDs for a CSP containing any nonsterile starting component.

15.1-22 Is a summary of the maximum BUD times available?

See **Exhibits 15-1** through **15-4** based on the CSP category and storage temperature.

EXHIBIT 15-1. Maximum BUDs for Category 1 CSPs

Category 1 CSP BUDs	
Controlled Room Temperature	Refrigerated
12 hours	24 hours

BUD = beyond-use date, CSP = compounded sterile preparation

EXHIBIT 15-2. Maximum BUDs for Aseptically-Prepared Category 2 CSPs with No Sterility Testing

Category 2 CSPs (aseptically-prepared, no sterility testing)			
	Controlled Room Temperature	Refrigerated	Frozen
Made from only sterile components	4 days	10 days	45 days
Including any nonsterile starting component	1 day	4 days	45 days

BUD = beyond-use date, CSP = compounded sterile preparation

EXHIBIT 15-3. Maximum BUDs for Aseptically-Prepared Category 2 CSPs with Sterility Test Passed

Category 2 CSPs (aseptically-prepared, sterility test passed)		
Controlled Room Temperature	Refrigerated	Frozen
30 days	45 days	60 days

BUD = beyond-use date, CSP = compounded sterile preparation

EXHIBIT 15-4. Maximum BUDs for Terminally-Sterilized Category 2 CSPs with No Sterility Testing

Category 2 CSPs (terminally-sterilized, no sterility test)		
Controlled Room Temperature	Refrigerated	Frozen
14 days	28 days	45 days

BUD = beyond-use date, CSP = compounded sterile preparation

EXHIBIT 15-5. Maximum BUDs for Terminally-Sterilized Category 2 CSPs with Sterility Test Passed

Category 2 CSPs (terminally-sterilized, sterility test passed)		
Controlled Room Temperature	Refrigerated	Frozen
45 days	60 days	90 days

BUD = beyond-use date, CSP = compounded sterile preparation

EXHIBIT 15-6. Maximum BUDs for Category 3 CSPs

Category 3 CSPs			
	Controlled Room Temperature	Refrigerated	Frozen
Aseptically prepared, sterility tested, passed all required tests for Category 3	60 days	90 days	120 days
Terminally sterilized, sterility tested, passed all required tests for Category 3	90 days	120 days	180 days

BUD = beyond-use date, CSP = compounded sterile preparation

15.1-23 We reconstitute and freeze some antibiotic syringes as Category 2 CSPs. Can I keep them for 45 days, then move them to the refrigerator for another 10 days?

No. BUDs are not additive. In this situation, the frozen syringes need to be discarded 45 days after compounding if not used (or earlier if they are not stable for that long).

15.1-24 We reconstitute and refrigerate some antibiotic syringes as Category 2 CSPs and have given them a 10-day BUD. If we take them out of the refrigerator on day 4, what is the room temperature BUD?

BUDs are not additive, so the maximum time you could use them for is 10 days refrigerated (if they are stable that long). In this situation, you could assign a room temperature stability of up to 4 days (if they are stable that long at room temperature). But, would you need to keep it at room temperature? Consider if it could be kept refrigerated until shortly before time of administration.

15.1-25 We warm some solutions (either before use or after compounding). What is the BUD for solutions placed in warmers?

You need to follow the manufacturer's information and place the solutions in a controlled temperature warmer. IV manufacturers have this information because surgical services often warm solutions.

15.1-26 Can I extend the BUDs beyond those listed in <797>?

Extending BUDs is only permitted if USP monographs are used or Category 3 requirements are met. (See <797> for complete information.[3]) To use the BUD in the USP monograph, the CSP must be compounded as directed, using the same packaging, the same storage temperature, and completion of any required testing. Category 3 requirements include additional facility and personnel requirements, environmental monitoring, and stability, sterility, and endotoxin testing.

15.1-27 I have published studies that have BUDs of 1 or 2 years. Can I use them?

No. Even if all Category 3 requirements are met, the BUD is limited to 60 to 180 days, depending on the type of preparation (aseptic or terminally sterilized) and the storage temperature. The only exception is for use of a USP monograph when the compounding exactly follows those instructions. See <797> for complete information.[3]

15.1-28 I have published studies that show 100% of the compound remaining on day 30. Can I extrapolate that information to use a longer BUD?

No, not without other information to support it. The authors may have stopped the study at day 30, so that's all they can report. Perhaps the compound is stable longer, but you have no proof of that.

15.1-29 Is it always OK to use the default dates listed in <797>?

No. These are not default dates; these are the maximum times allowed. Other factors may require you to use shorter times, including the following:

▶ How the CSP reacts over time
▶ The interaction of the container or closure with the CSP
▶ Microbial growth

15.1-30 If I make a CSP today, does the time for the BUD start today or tomorrow?

The BUD begins from the time the preparation is started.

15.1-31 Do BUDs for intrathecal or epidural CSPs need to be less than those defaults listed in <797>?

<797> does not distinguish among any specific sterile dosage form. However, many organizations use BUDs shorter than the allowable defaults, especially for dosage forms that are administered as intraspinal or ophthalmic drugs.

15.1-32 Pharmacy references often have stability information that is longer than the BUDs allowed in <797>. Can I use the references?

There are several valuable references often used, including *ASHP Injectable Drug Information 2023*,[46] Simpson/Schaefer's *Extended Stability for Parenteral Drugs*,[47] and King's *Guide to Parenteral Admixtures*.[48] These are references for stability. You need to use the *shorter* of stability (such as from the manufacturer, these references, or other peer-reviewed sources) or sterility limits as defined in <797> BUD tables.

15.1-33 My state has the old BUDs in regulations. Do I follow them or new <797> information?

Use the more conservative of the times.

15.1-34 Do the BUDs in <797> apply to compounds made for animals?

Yes. <797> applies to both human and animal nonsterile compounds. There is no distinction among species for BUD assignment.

15.1-35 Does the BUD differ based on the category of compound (low, medium, or high risk)?

The risk categories were in the 2008 version of <797> and are no longer used. The 2022 version of <797> uses Categories 1, 2, and 3 to distinguish the allowable BUDs.

15.2 ACTIVE PHARMACEUTICAL INGREDIENTS AND OTHER COMPONENTS

15.2-1 What is the BUD of opened jars of components?

Active pharmaceutical ingredients (APIs) need to come from an FDA-registered supplier so they will have an expiration date assigned by the manufacturer. For components without an expiration date, mark the date when they are received, and assign a BUD no longer than 1 year from the date of receipt.

15.2-2 What should I do with old bottles of chemicals and other components?

Properly discard them.

15.2-3 Can the container used for the package of a CSP affect the stability?

Yes. Both the container and the closure used can affect stability.

15.3 VIAL/BAG SYSTEMS

15.3-1 What is the BUD of products like ADD-Vantage™, MiniBag Plus, VIAL-MATE, addEASE®, and similar systems?

If these are attached and activated on the patient care unit, they need to be used right away.

If the vials and bags are attached (docked), but not activated and will be stored for future use, it is considered compounding, so the personnel, facility, and other requirements of <797> must be met. Note that not all bag/vial systems are approved for docking, storage, and future use. For those that are approved for docking and future use, the BUD is not limited to the times in the default tables because manufacturers perform testing on these prior to Food and Drug Administration (FDA) approval. You can use the BUDs provided by the manufacturer that are based on the bag component remaining with the specifications for the fluid in the plastic container.

15.4 VIALS AND OTHER DOSAGE FORMS

15.4-1 Do BUDs apply to manufactured products, or only compounded preparations?

They apply to vials and other manufactured components if they are used on more than one occasion.

15.4-2 What is the BUD of a single-dose ampule?

A single-dose ampule must be discarded immediately after use.

15.4-3 What's the BUD of a single-dose vial?

If a single-dose vial is opened or punctured in ambient air, it must be discarded immediately after use. If a single-dose vial is opened or punctured in ISO 5 or cleaner air (such as inside a PEC), it may be used for up to 12 hours as long as the storage requirements from the manufacturer are followed.

15.4-4 Is a manufactured IV bag (like a saline bag used for reconstituting antibiotics) a single-dose or a multiple-dose container?

It is a single-dose container. If a parenteral container intended for single use is opened or punctured in ISO 5 or cleaner air (such as inside a primary engineering control [PEC]), it may be used for up to 12 hours as long as the storage requirements from the manufacturer are followed.

15.4-5 Once an IV is spiked, what is the BUD?

Once an IV is spiked, it should be used right away.

15.4-6 Is the BUD of a manufactured solution different from a compounded CSP?

Spiking and hanging a manufactured IV solution is not compounding, so <797> does not apply. You can use the manufacturer's expiration date, as long as the produce has been stored according to the manufacturer's instructions (e.g., proper temperature, intact packaging).

15.4-7 What's the BUD of an IV made during a code?

A CSP made at bedside during a code would be used right away. It needs to follow the immediate-use information in <797>.

15.4-8 When I go in the operating room (OR) prep room on evenings, I see several cases of IV solutions spiked and hanging. The OR says this is standard practice and there is no BUD. Is this correct?

This is not specifically addressed in <797> but is an issue of safe practice. Once an IV is spiked, it should be used right away. There are no preservatives in the solution.

Your infection preventionist can help you eliminate this unsafe practice. Also see the Association for Professionals in Infection Control and Epidemiology (APIC) position paper *Safe Injection, Infusion, and Medication Vial Practices in Health Care*[26] for further information.

15.4-9 Is a manufactured irrigation bottle a single-dose or a multiple-dose container?

It is a single-dose container.

15.4-10 What is the BUD of a multiple-dose vial?

It is 28 days unless otherwise specified in the product labeling.

15.4-11 Once punctured, should a multiple-dose vial be refrigerated or kept in the hood?

This is a stability, sterility, and patient safety issue. You need to follow the manufacturer's instructions for storage, including BUD and storage temperature. The Institute for Safe Medication Practices (ISMP) has safety information about the risk of storing vials inside a PEC that are not being used for the preparation being mixed.[33] Establish your policy with all these issues in mind.

15.4-12 If I am going to save a multiple-dose vial for future use, do I need to date it with the open date or the end date?

You need to date it with the BUD. Your policy may specify additional requirements.

15.4-13 If a multiple-dose vial is missing the cap, does that affect the BUD?

Vial caps are dust covers for the stopper; they do not indicate a sterile septum. If you can be sure the vial has not been compromised, there is no difference if it has a cap or not. If this occurs more than rarely, it either needs to be reported to the FDA MedWatch program[49] if received from the supplier, or investigated thoroughly if it emanates from your storage area. It could be related to tampering of the drugs.

15.4-14 What is the BUD of a pharmacy bulk package (PBP)?

PBPs are single-dose vials containing many doses (e.g., a 10-g cefazolin vial or a 50-mL vial of an electrolyte intended for total parenteral nutrition [TPN] compounding). The PBP will have a BUD time in the product labeling that must be followed. PBPs may only be opened or punctured under ISO 5 or cleaner air (e.g., inside a PEC).

15.4-15 If a PBP is labeled with a manufacturer's in-use time of 4 hours, can I still use it for 12 hours since I opened it under the hood?

No. You need to follow the information in the product labeling.

15.5 COMPOUNDED STOCK BAGS

15.5-1 We mix an electrolyte bag to use in neonatal TPNs. How long is the bag good for?

There are a lot of different situations when stock bags are prepared, so be sure to refer to the full text in <797> for your specific situation. A common situation is preparing a stock bag in a cleanroom suite, adding one or more conventionally manufactured electrolytes into a manufactured IV solution. Once you mix the bag, you can store it (unused) for up to the allowed BUD based on the storage temperature. That could be as long as 10 days refrigerated for Category 2 CSPs if the mixture is stable that long. When you need to use it, puncture it inside the ISO 5 PEC and use it for up to 12 hours (or it's assigned BUD, whichever is shorter) then discard it.

The CSPs made from that stock bag could potentially have a BUD that is *no longer* than the BUD on the stock bag. For example, if your stock bag has a BUD of 10 days and you remove it from the refrigerator on day 5, the CSPs made with it could have a BUD of 4 days (if stable that long). If you remove the stock bag and puncture it on day 7, the CSPs made from it could have a BUD of 3 days (if stable that long). However, consider a more conservative approach, such as mixing smaller stock bags and using a shorter BUD. Many organizations mix a stock bag, use it that day (within 12 hours), and use a short BUD for the subsequently mixed CSPs, such as 24 hours.

15.5-2 Our 503B outsourcing facility mixes stock bags for us. Do they have a different BUD than if I mixed them myself?

Find out if your outsourcing facility has validated studies to support a BUD beyond which you would use. Make your decision on that, coupled with the requirements in <797>.

DISPENSING AND PACKAGING *16*

16.1 What are some key issues to confirm when dispensing a compounded sterile preparation?

Check that the compounded sterile preparation (CSP) matches the order or prescription, the master formulation record (MFR), and the compounding record (CR), and check that it is labeled correctly. If the CSP was compounded in advance of dispensing, a visual check needs to be done to be sure it still meets the physical appearance expected. If the MFR requires specific testing (such as pH), be sure that is done and recorded.

16.2 What has to be on the label of a compounded sterile preparation?

The label on the immediate container must display at least the following:

▶ Assigned internal identification number (such as barcode, prescription or order number, or lot number)
▶ Active ingredients, including amount/activity or concentration
▶ Dosage form
▶ Amount or volume in the container if not obvious
▶ Storage temperature if other than controlled room temperature
▶ Beyond-use date
▶ If it is a single-dose container, a statement stating that when space permits
▶ If it is a multiple-dose container, a statement stating exactly that

The labeling on the CSP should include the following:

▶ Indication that the preparation is compounded
▶ Route of administration
▶ Any special handling instructions
▶ Any applicable warning statements
▶ Name, address, and contact information of the compounding facility if the CSP will be sent outside the facility or healthcare system where it was compounded

Your state board or accreditation organization may have additional requirements.

16.3 What's the difference between the label and the labeling?

The *label* needs to be affixed to the final container. *Labeling* includes the label and any additional information except the outer shipping container.

DOI 10.37573/9781585287260.016

16.4   Why would there be a different spot to put a label on a CSP?

The distinction between label and labeling is to allow for situations where the immediate container is too small for the entire labeling requirements. For example, you might make several 1-mL syringes or eye drops in small containers. Each dose needs to have the label requirements, but the rest of the information could be on a bag in which the syringes or eye drop bottles are placed.

16.5   Does a CSP label have to include the fact that it is compounded?

<797> says the labeling should include the fact that the preparation is compounded. Your state may have more stringent requirements.

16.6   Does the technician who mixed the CSP and the pharmacist who checked the CSP need to initial the label?

Define that in your policies and procedures. Ideally, an image of the label with that information (initialed either manually or electronically) would be available. But many organizations do not yet have the technology to support permanent electronic capture of that information. You need to have a method to identify the individuals involved in the compounding process and the person who verified the final CSP. That information needs to be on the CR and retrievable after the CSP has been discarded.

16.7   Are there requirements for the packaging that must be used for CSPs that are mailed or shipped?

Your policies need to define how you will appropriately package CSPs that will be mailed or shipped. The packaging needs to be able to protect the integrity of the CSP and the safety of personnel who handle them.

16.8   Are temperature monitors required for CSPs that are shipped?

You need to determine that based on the CSP and shipping process.

CLEANING AND DISINFECTING *17*

17.1 GENERAL INFORMATION

17.1-1 What is the difference between deactivating, decontaminating, cleaning, and disinfecting?

▶ *Deactivating* renders a substance inert.

▶ *Decontaminating* removes substances from the surface using a disposable wiper.

▶ *Cleaning* removes residue such as dirt from surfaces using a cleaning agent and manual process.

▶ *Disinfecting* is then done to ensure the surfaces are free from contamination.

17.1-2 <800> mentions decontaminating, but <797> doesn't. Why? Do I still need to decontaminate my chemo areas?

Yes. You need to decontaminate areas where hazardous drugs are handled. Decontamination isn't mentioned in <797> because all hazardous drug handling needs to comply with both <797> and <800>. See <800>[4] for those details.

17.1-3 Why are sporicidals used?

These agents destroy spores when applied at an appropriate concentration for the contact (dwell) time listed in the product labeling.

17.1-4 Which is done first: cleaning or disinfecting?

Cleaning is done first, followed by disinfecting surfaces. An Environmental Protection Agency (EPA)-registered one-step disinfectant cleaner may be able to be used according to the manufacturer's instructions to perform both steps in one application.

17.1-5 Do I need to wear garb when cleaning?

Yes. Cleaning inside the sterile compounding area requires the same garb as when compounding. In some cases, additional eye and respiratory protection may be needed. Many organizations include goggles to protect eyes when cleaning agents are used above waist level. Check the manufacturer's information for the solutions you are using for additional information specific to that chemical.

DOI 10.37573/9781585287260.017

17.1-6 What does *dwell time* mean?

Dwell time is the amount of time a solution needs to be wet and in contact with the surface to meet the product claims. The dwell time for EPA-registered one-step disinfectant cleaning solutions is listed on the product labeling. Because of the air flow in the PECs and compounding suites, a long dwell time is impractical; the agent won't stay wet for the required time. A required dwell time more than 3 minutes may be impractical.

17.1-7 We always clean with sterile alcohol. Is that enough?

No. Alcohol is not a cleaner; it is a sanitizing agent. You need to use an agent that contains a detergent or surfactant to clean.

17.1-8 Is alcohol a disinfectant or a sanitizing agent?

It is a sanitizing agent unless the brand used is EPA-registered and the dwell time is followed. Some brands are labeled as disinfectants but require a specific dwell time of 5 to 10 minutes. Alcohol won't stay wet that long in most situations in an IV room because of the air flow.

17.1-9 Can an ultraviolet light be used to sanitize an area?

It cannot be used instead of 70% sterile isopropyl alcohol (sIPA).

7.1-10 Is sterile alcohol required in <797>?

Yes. When alcohol is used in or on the PEC or containers being placed in the PEC, 70% sterile isopropyl alcohol is required.

17.1-11 Should cleaning agents be rotated?

There is no requirement to rotate agents to combat the development of microbial resistance. Bactericidal cleaning agents are used as daily cleaners, but a sporicidal cleaning agent must be used monthly. This is not rotation per se; the selection of a different agent is based on the different mechanism of action.

17.1-12 Are reusable mops acceptable to use?

They are not prohibited, but consider the process you use. Standardizing on disposable mop heads removes the concern of spreading contamination from one area to another.

17.1-13 What is the best way to monitor that cleaning has been done?

The designated person should monitor that this is done. Cleaning done daily or less frequently needs to be documented. Some state regulations require additional or more frequent documentation.

17.1-14 Do pharmacy personnel need to do all the cleaning of sterile compounding areas?

Only compounders with documented competence in sterile compounding can clean PECs and other sensitive equipment. Either pharmacy or environmental services staff can clean the rooms, but any personnel involved in cleaning sterile compounding areas needs to have documented competency. Regulators and accreditation organizations often expect pharmacy staff to oversee the training and confirm the competence of nonpharmacy personnel who clean sterile compounding areas.

17.1-15 When and with what do supplies going into the sterile compounding area need to be cleaned?

Your policies and procedures need to detail how the outside of containers (e.g., vials, boxes in which vials are packaged) are cleaned prior to placement in a sterile compounding area. Drugs and supplies going into the buffer room or crossing over the perimeter line in an SCA must first be wiped with a sporicidal agent or a sterile disinfectant like sIPA. Immediately prior to placing drugs and other supplies in the PEC, the outside of each item must be wiped with sIPA. For supplies such as syringes that are received in sterile packaging, the outside of the package needs to be wiped; the sterile syringes inside the package do not need to be wiped if the package is opened as they are placed inside the PEC.

17.1-16 What is a one-step cleaner? Can I use these in the intravenous (IV) room?

Yes, you can. An EPA-registered one-step disinfectant cleaner means that both cleaning and disinfecting occur in one step. These solutions are not appropriate when dirty areas are cleaned, but that should not be an issue in a sterile compounding area other than cleaning on commissioning the area.

17.1-17 What cleaning and disinfecting needs to be done daily?

Daily cleaning and disinfecting needs to include the following:

▶ PEC
▶ Equipment inside PEC
▶ Surface of the removable work tray of the PEC
▶ Pass-through chambers
▶ Work surfaces outside the PEC but inside the SEC
▶ Surfaces of sinks

Floors need to be cleaned daily but do not have to be disinfected with sIPA.

17.1-18 Does the PEC need to be cleaned and disinfected every 30 minutes?

The PEC surface needs to be wiped with sIPA at least every 30 minutes if compounding takes less than 30 minutes. If compounding takes longer than 30 minutes, wipe the work surface after compounding is completed.

17.1-19 What cleaning needs to be done weekly?

There is no specific weekly cleaning required in <797> for Category 1 or 2, but many organizations identify specific areas (for which <797> requires monthly cleaning) to be cleaned weekly. If you require that, be sure your procedures and logs accurately reflect that.

Additional cleaning for rooms used to prepare Category 3 is required at least weekly when compounding occurs in those rooms. A sporicidal disinfectant needs to be applied to surfaces in rooms used for Category 3 compounding, including:

▸ All interior surfaces of the PEC and any equipment in the PEC

▸ Removable work tray of the PEC

▸ Pass-through chambers

▸ Work surfaces outside the PEC

▸ Floors

17.1-20 What cleaning needs to be done monthly?

For rooms used to prepare Category 1 or Category 2 CSPs, a sporicidal disinfectant must be used at least monthly. Surfaces to be cleaned include the following:

▸ All interior surfaces of the PEC and equipment within the PEC (*note:* monthly cleaning and disinfecting inside the PEC is always at least two steps)

　▲ Application of an EPA-registered one-step sporicidal disinfectant cleaner, then

　▲ Wiping with sIPA after the cleaning agent dwell time has been achieved

▸ Cleaning, disinfecting, and application of a sporicidal underneath the removable worktray of the PEC

▸ Work surfaces outside the PEC

▸ Pass-through chambers

▸ Floors

▸ Sinks

▸ Walls

▸ Doors and door frames

▸ Ceiling in the compounding suite

　▲ <797> allows ceilings in segregated compounding areas to be cleaned, disinfected, and applied with a sporicidal when visibly soiled or when contamination is known or suspected. However, consider performing this monthly.

▸ Storage shelving, bins, and their contents

▸ Equipment used outside the PEC but within the SEC

▸ All surfaces of pass-throughs

▸ All surfaces of PECs and any furniture (e.g., tables, shelves, carts)

17.1-21 If my IV room isn't used every day, do I still need to clean it every day?

No. Daily cleaning does not have to be done on days the room is not used. However, even if you left the room clean on the last day it was used, the chapter requires you to perform daily cleaning before resuming sterile compounding. If the sterile compounding area isn't used in a month, then perform the daily and monthly cleaning requirements prior to compounding. Your state board may have more stringent requirements.

17.1-22 Are there requirements for who can clean the IV room?

Yes. Only compounding personnel with documented competence in performing hand hygiene and garbing appropriate to the space as well as in performing cleaning activities can clean the PECs. Either pharmacy personnel or environmental services personnel can clean the SECs. Environmental services personnel do not need to perform gloved fingertip and thumb sampling, because they don't compound, but they do need to complete the other garbing and hand hygiene competencies. The designated person should oversee the competency requirements for any personnel outside the pharmacy as well as all compounding personnel.

17.1-23 How often does competency documentation for cleaning need to occur?

For personnel who clean but do not compound, documentation is required initially and then as often is defined by organizational policy. (Most organizations have an annual competency review.) Competency for cleaning (knowledge of solutions and preparation, processes to use, garb, etc.) must be consistent for both pharmacy and environmental personnel. Be sure to document any in-services throughout the year that deal with cleaning and, if personnel outside the pharmacy clean the SECs, be sure to include them in the in-servicing as well.

17.1-24 How should the IV room be cleaned after a power outage?

There is no specific information in <797>, so your procedure needs to be part of your organizational policies. The approach some organizations have taken include differentiating the duration of the outage. For example, if the outage is very brief (for example, no more than a few minutes), cleaning the PEC may be sufficient. If the outage is a bit longer, but no more than an hour, perform a daily clean of the PEC and SEC. If the outage is greater than an hour, a more detailed cleaning process is needed since there would not have been the appropriate air flow into the space. Consider either using a bacteriocidal twice and a sporicidal, or a bacteriocidal and two applications of a sporicidal.

17.2 TYPES OF CLEANING SOLUTIONS

17.2-1 How do I know what cleaning solutions to select?

Sterile 70% isopropyl alcohol must be used to wipe inside the PECs after cleaning has been performed. Select your decontamination and cleaning solutions by evaluating the availability (which may be related to your buying group options), safety (for both personnel and your surfaces), and effectiveness.[50] Your infection control practitioner may be able to help with identifying appropriate solutions. Consider use of ready-to-use solutions rather than those you must dilute. The EPA-registered one-step disinfectant cleaners will have compatibility and contact time information.

17.2-2 How do I know I am using the correct dilutions of cleaning solutions?

Read the manufacturer's instructions. Ready-to-use solutions are the most convenient because they do not require dilution. Be sure that the solutions remain in contact with the surface for the appropriate contact (dwell) time. Use cleaning and decontaminating agents for which the manufacturers specify dwell time or contact time in their instructions for use.

17.2-3 Is sterile water a cleaning solution?

No. Water is not a cleaner but may be used to dissolve residue in the PEC.

17.2-4 Is bleach a cleaning solution?

Not as a single agent. It is a sporicidal (when used in the appropriate concentration for the appropriate dwell time) but needs to be partnered with a surfactant or detergent to be considered a cleaner.

17.2-5 If bleach is used as a sporicidal agent, what strength should be used?

It needs to be at least 0.5% which is often listed on products as 5,000 parts per million. The concentration can be found on the product labeling. However, because bleach is often diluted, be sure the final concentration doesn't fall below 0.5%.

17.2-6 Once bleach is diluted, how long is it good for?

It needs to be mixed daily.

17.2-7 Are ready-to-use solutions required?

They aren't required by <797>, but they are desirable. Ready-to-use products are already properly diluted, so provide a safe process for both patients (the concentration is correct) and personnel (because they don't have to mix potentially dangerous chemicals). If you use a concentrate mixed with water, this process must be documented each time a solution is mixed. Measuring devices must be provided and properly maintained. Sterile Water for Irrigation is needed as the diluent if the resulting solution will be used inside of the PEC.

17.2-8 How should cleaning agents be applied?

It's best to apply the solutions to a disposable wiper or cleaning tool cover. Never spray into the HEPA filters and never in hazardous drug preparation areas. In many cases, you will also need tools to reach the areas you need to clean. The reusable tool handles and holders need to be dedicated for use in the sterile compounding area; for hazardous drug rooms (buffer rooms and containment segregated compounding area [C-SCAs]), dedicate reusable tool handles and holders to only that area. The tool handles and holders need to be cleanable and cleaned and disinfected before and after each use. They cannot be made of wood or other particle-shedding material.

17.2-9 Can any type of cloth be used for the wiper?

No. Wipers need to be disposable and low-linting.

17.2-10 Do cleaning products have to be sterile?

Any solution used inside the PEC needs to be sterile.

17.3 CLEANING PECs AND OTHER COMPOUNDING EQUIPMENT

17.3-1 How often should PECs and other equipment used for compounding be cleaned?

Any equipment used to compound should be cleaned as soon as possible once compounding is completed.

17.3-2 What types of solutions should be used for cleaning the hoods?

For PECs used for nonhazardous compounding, two steps are necessary:

1. Clean with a detergent, then
2. Wipe with sterile 70% IPA

For PECs used for hazardous drug compounding, three steps are necessary:

1. Decontaminate with an agent that has been verified to decontaminate HDs, then
2. Clean with a detergent, then
3. Wipe with sterile 70% IPA

You may need to use sterile water to remove visible particles prior to the cleaning step if debris or residue is present.

17.3-3 What does *terminal cleaning* mean?

It is not a term used in <797> nor an adequate description of the required process. (It comes from a patient care perspective; sterile compounding is a different process.) What is generally meant by this is the weekly or the monthly cleaning and that is the term that should be used.

17.3-4 Who should clean the hoods?

Only compounding personnel may decontaminate, clean, and disinfect the PECs and the equipment in them.

17.3-5 How often do the hoods or other compounding surfaces need to be cleaned during compounding?

Cleaning and sanitizing are different actions. First, the inside of PECs must be sanitized with sIPA at the beginning and end of each shift, after spills, and when surface contamination is known or suspected. The deck (flat surface) of the hood and work surfaces need to be sanitized between compounding CSPs with different components and more frequently if needed.

Cleaning and disinfection must be performed daily at the end of the compounding day (or at a defined time during the day if the sterile compounding area is used 24/7).

17.3-6 Do I have to clean the hoods even on days they are not used?

No. If the hood has not been used in more than 24 hours, then <797> says it must be cleaned and disinfected with a cleaning agent and then wiped with sterile IPA before use. If it was cleaned and less than 24 hours has elapsed, wipe all surfaces inside the hood with sIPA before use. Your policies and procedures need to reflect your actual process. If the hood is turned off or power is lost for any reason, then the daily cleaning and disinfection must be performed before it is used for sterile compounding. Your state board may have more stringent requirements.

17.3-7 How often does an automated compounding device need to be cleaned?

At least daily when it (or the PEC in which it resides) is cleaned. It may need to be cleaned more frequently if source containers spill on the components. Remember that this equipment is inside or close to the direct compounding area and must be wiped with sIPA as frequently as the PEC deck is wiped.

17.3-8 How often does a repeater pump need to be cleaned?

At least daily when it (or the PEC in which it resides) is cleaned. It may need to be cleaned more frequently if source containers spill on the components. Remember that this equipment is inside or close to the direct compounding area and must be wiped with sIPA as frequently as the PEC deck is wiped.

17.3-9 How often does any computer equipment need to be cleaned?

At least daily when it (or the PEC in which it resides) is cleaned. It may need to be cleaned more frequently if there are spills or drips on the components. Remember that this equipment is inside or close to the direct compounding area and must be wiped with sIPA as frequently as the PEC deck is wiped.

17.3-10 If the power goes off, do we need to clean the hoods?

Yes. Anytime power is lost to a PEC or is turned off all interior surfaces of the PEC and anything residing on the PEC deck must be cleaned and disinfected with an EPA-registered one-step sporicidal cleaner and then those surfaces wiped with sIPA after the dwell time of the sporicidal has been achieved. Define that in your policies and procedures.

17.3-11 Do we need to clean syringes as we take them out of the packages?

No. Sterile supplies in sterile packaging do not need to be cleaned as long as the outside of the packages are clean and they are opened inside the PEC.

17.3-12 How long can a bottle of sterile alcohol be used?

After opening sterile solutions and supplies, the container can be used as specified by the manufacturer and listed in the organization's policies. For example, a bottle of sterile alcohol or a package of sterile wipers can be opened in ISO 5 and remain there as long as not prohibited by the manufacturer and defined in your policy.

17.4 CLEANING COMPOUNDING AREAS

17.4-1 Is it OK for environmental services personnel to clean the floors while we are compounding?

No. Cleaning cannot occur while you are compounding.

17.4-2 Is alcohol sufficient to clean the compounding areas?

No. Alcohol is neither a decontaminating agent nor a cleaner. Alcohol is a disinfectant when it is registered with the EPA and the dwell time listed is used. Use sIPA after cleaning has occurred inside PECs.

17.4-3 Who should clean the compounding area?

Either compounding personnel or environmental services personnel can clean the compounding area floors, walls, and ceilings. Training and documented competence is required. In any case, all compounding personnel should be competent in this task in case environmental services personnel are not available. Regulatory agencies and accreditation organizations often expect pharmacy to oversee the competency of nonpharmacy employees who clean the compounding area.

17.4-4 What is a "high-touch" area?

Areas that are frequently touched, like carts, counters, refrigerators, pass-throughs, door handles, etc.

17.4-5 Do I have to clean the compounding area even on days it is not used?

No, but be sure to clean the hood and compounding areas before you begin compounding. Your state board may have more stringent requirements. Your policies and procedures need to reflect your actual process.

17.4-6 How often does the office space inside the anteroom need to be cleaned?

If you mean a counter where staging of supplies occurs, that needs to be cleaned at least daily. If you mean space for administrative activities, that should not be occurring in the anteroom or buffer room. If you perform activities that could be done outside the sterile compounding area, take steps to improve that process and in the meantime, clean more frequently than required.

17.4-7 How often do pass-through chambers need to be cleaned?

Daily.

17.4-8 How often do refrigerators in the sterile compounding area need to be cleaned?

As often as necessary to keep them clean. Also perform viable air sampling near them to ensure they are not compromising your microbial state of control.

17.4-9 Because I compound only occasionally, do I have to clean my whole pharmacy with the same frequency as the compounding area?

<797> deals only with sterile compounding. Your state board regulations may have additional information.

17.4-10 How often should I use alcohol to clean the floor?

Alcohol is *not* a cleaner; it is a sanitizing/disinfecting agent. There is no value in using alcohol or sterile alcohol for this purpose. Use a detergent and disinfectant to clean the floor.

17.4-11 Can the IV room floor be stripped and re-waxed?

No; there should not be wax on the floor at all. Floors must be smooth and sealed with continuous, welded seams. Epoxy floors are common. Another option is sheet vinyl or rubber products that are designed for use in cleanroom-type areas. Any floor surface must be able to withstand frequent cleaning with the solutions used (disinfectants, sporicidals, etc.).

17.5 CLEANING SUPPLIES NEEDED FOR COMPOUNDING

17.5-1 When and with what should drug vials, IV bags, needles, and syringes be cleaned?

This is a process involving several steps. If a hazardous drug is received (all NIOSH Table 1 antineoplastics[19] and any other National Institute for Occupational Safety and Health (NIOSH) hazardous drugs that have not been entity-exempt in the organization's Assessment of Risk need to be wiped prior to the location where they will be stored. For NIOSH Table 1 antineoplastic drugs, you should be receiving the drugs enclosed in impervious plastic within the tote or other shipping container. See <800>[4] and *The Chapter <800> Answer Book*[9] for information.

For nonhazardous drugs and supplies, use the following steps:

1. Prior to taking drugs, IVs, and other supplies into the clean side of the anteroom, into pass-throughs, or inside the perimeter of the SCA or C-SCA, wipe the outside of the package with a sporicidal agent, EPA-registered disinfectant, or sIPA. Be sure that the process you use does not obliterate any labeling on the product, such as lot number and expiration date.

2. Immediately before the drugs, IVs, or supplies are placed in the PEC, wipe the outside of the vial, IV bag or overwrap, outside of the packaging of sterile supplies, or other component with sIPA. Be sure not to saturate the packaging. Allow the sIPA to dry. Do not wipe the syringes, needles, IV sets, and other sterile components that come packaged as sterile items as long as the package is opened inside the PEC.

3. Critical sites (vial stoppers, necks of ampules, IV bag ports, etc.) exposed in the PEC must be wiped with sIPA before puncturing or entering the component.

ENVIRONMENTAL MONITORING *18*

18.1 GENERAL INFORMATION

18.1-1 What is environmental monitoring?

Environmental monitoring (EM) is the process by which facilities are evaluated and tested to ensure maintenance of a state of control. In <797>, it concerns viable monitoring.

18.1-2 Is environmental monitoring the same as certification?

No. They are different. *Certification* is the process of validating the nonviable elements of your PEC and SEC, including particle counts, air flow and pattern evaluation, pressure gradients, and other parameters that a compounding area is expected to maintain. *Environmental monitoring* is the testing and evaluation of viable (bacterial and fungal) sources of potential contamination.

18.1-3 Our environmental monitoring is done by our certifier. Is that OK?

You, your certifier, or other qualified personnel can perform the monitoring.

18.1-4 Does our environmental monitoring have to be done by our certifier?

No. It can be done by you, your certifier, or other qualified personnel.

18.1-5 What does viable monitoring do?

It detects microbial contamination.

18.1-6 I thought only the certifier could do air sampling. Is that correct?

No. It can be done by you, your certifier, or other qualified personnel. An independent certifier needs to certify your primary engineering controls (PECs) and secondary engineering controls (SECs), and that includes air sampling for particles. The air and surface sampling done for viable environmental monitoring is different.

18.1-7 Do I need a detailed policy, or can I depend on what my certifier does?

Certification checks nonviable elements; environmental monitoring is different. Your certifier may perform environmental monitoring for you, but you need to provide the certifier with your policies and monitoring plan.

DOI 10.37573/9781585287260.018

18.1-8 Do hoods and rooms need to be tested before they are used?

Yes. Hoods and rooms must be tested and acceptable results returned. This is part of the commissioning of the area. You need to be sure your PECs and SECs are in a state of control prior to using them for sterile compounding.

18.1-9 How often does environmental monitoring need to be done?

Electronic air sampling by impaction and surface sampling must be done initially to establish baseline levels of quality and to be sure the area is in a state of control. Following the commissioning of your sterile compounding area, electronic air sampling must be done at least every 6 months and surface sampling must be done at least monthly for Category 1 and 2. For Category 3, there are requirements to check air within 30 days prior to the start of mixing Category 3 CSPs. Following that, monthly sampling is required. Category 3 also requires weekly surface sampling and additional testing for batches and self-enclosed robots.

Any out of specification results (above the action level) need to be supplemented by follow-up monitoring if your areas show growth above the action level or when you want to trend the results for more robust monitoring.

18.1-10 What does *commissioning* mean?

Commissioning means checking your sterile compounding area prior to compounding in that area to be sure the space is in a state of control: the PECs and SECs are operating correctly, all equipment has undergone checks required by the manufacturer's specifications, there is no concerning microbial contamination in the area, etc.

18.1-11 What is a sampling plan?

The sampling plan is your policy and procedure that details what samples will be taken, what media will be used, how the samples will be incubated, how the incubator temperature is controlled and monitoring, how action levels will be addressed, and other details that will allow you to assess the state of control of the sterile compounding area.

18.1-12 What is an action level?

An action level is the level above which you need to take action. The action taken is intended to correct the reason you had microbial growth.

18.1-13 What is an alert level?

Alert levels aren't defined in <797>, but you may want to set an alert level, which needs to be lower than the action level, to indicate a trigger for specific requirements in your monitoring policy.

18.1-14 What are highly pathogenic organisms?

Highly pathogenic organisms are any organism that could be an issue to a susceptible patient. This term was used in previous versions of <797> but is not in the 2023 revision.

18.1-15 What is a CFU?

A CFU is a colony-forming unit. Each distinct colony on a media plate is 1 CFU.

18.1-16 Do I have to test for fungus if I don't make any high-risk preparations?

Yes. There is no longer the distinction based on risk level. The 2023 revision removed that and replaced it with Category 1, 2, and 3. Air and surface sampling needs to test for both bacteria and fungus.

18.1-17 Do I have to incubate the samples?

Yes. The samples need to be incubated at a controlled temperature in an incubator.

18.1-18 Do I need an incubator in the pharmacy?

You need to be sure the samples are appropriately incubated. That might be done in your department (although do not place the incubator in the sterile compounding area), by your laboratory, or by an outside laboratory (which may be contracted by you or your certifier).

18.1-19 Is a warmer OK to use to incubate the samples?

No. You need to use an incubator.

18.1-20 Can I use the mannitol warmer to incubate the samples?

No. You need to use an incubator to incubate the samples at the temperature required in <797>. You certainly don't want to mix drugs with samples of growth media in the same device.

18.1-21 Does the incubator need special controls?

The device needs to be intended for use in incubating growth media. The temperature must be maintained and documented via continuous recording (preferred) or manually. The incubator must be outside the sterile compounding area and should be attached to emergency power.

18.1-22 Can the microbiology laboratory at the hospital incubate the samples?

They may be able to incubate the surface samples but probably not the air samples. Hospital laboratories are set up to handle patient samples, not environmental samples. Keep in mind that many have limited resources, so may not be able to take on the additional burden and may not have incubator space. If incubator space is the only issue, consider purchasing the incubator for the microbiology department to use for pharmacy samples.

18.1-23 Can an outside laboratory incubate the samples?

Yes, and this is often done by certifiers. The laboratory should be accredited to ISO 17025, which is the standard used by testing and calibration laboratories. The chain of custody of the samples is important to maintain.

18.1-24 Who should identify the growth?

A qualified individual such as a microbiologist.

18.1-25 Can I incubate the samples in the pharmacy and send them to the laboratory for identification?

Discuss this with your microbiology department. In some organizations, the incubator for the samples is stored in the pharmacy department but not in the sterile compounding area. If growth is found, a microbiologist could identify the organisms. The chain of custody for the samples is important to maintain.

18.1-26 Can I incubate the samples in the pharmacy and identify them myself?

The identification of microorganisms needs to be done with the assistance of a microbiologist. See *USP General Chapter <1113> Microbial Characterization, Identification, and Strain Typing.*[51] The chain of custody for the samples is important to maintain.

18.1-27 Does it really matter what is growing or is just the fact that there are a lot of CFUs on the plate enough information?

If the action level is exceeded, you need to attempt to identify the microorganism to the genus level with the assistance of a microbiologist.

18.1-28 What does *TNTC* mean on my microbiology report?

TNTC means too numerous to count. A report of TNTC is clearly above the action level.

18.2 ACTIVE AIR SAMPLING

18.2-1 What does *active air sampling* mean?

Use of an electronic sampling method that is done by impaction. A measured volume of air is drawn into a device that contains an agar plate. Any microbial contamination will be captured on the plate, which is then incubated.

18.2-2 What device is used to sample the air?

A microbial air sampler is the device used.

18.2-3 What is measured by active air sampling?

Microbial contamination in the PEC and SEC.

18.2-4 What has to be sampled?

Any ISO-classified space: all PECs, compounding suites (both anterooms and buffer rooms), and any high efficiency particulate air (HEPA)-filtered pass-through chamber.

18.2-5 How often is active air sampling required?

Initially to established baseline levels of quality and to be sure the area is in a state of control. Then, the minimum frequency is every 6 months for Category 1 and 2. (If your certifier does this for you, it will likely be done at the same time as the certification of the PECs and SECs.) Category 3 requires active air sampling initially prior to starting Category 3, then monthly. If growth above the action level is found, you will need to sample after remediation to be sure whatever caused the excursion has been corrected.

18.2-6 Do settling plates comply with <797>?

No. Settling plates are a passive test. You need to use active air sampling to comply with <797>.

18.2-7 Do I have to sample the air in pass-throughs?

If it is a HEPA-filtered pass-through, it needs to be sampled because it is an ISO classified area.

18.2-8 What media is used?

A general microbiological growth media that supports the growth of both bacteria and fungi must be used. Most organizations use trypticase soy agar (TSA) for detection of both. Some use TSA to detect bacteria and use a separate plate to detect fungus (with a media such as malt extract agar [MEA] or Sabouraud dextrose agar [SDA]).

See Box 5 in Section 6.2.2 of <797>[3] for detailed information.

18.2-9 What is the temperature required for incubators?

Two temperature ranges are required: 30–35°C, then 20–25°C. Some organizations use one incubator and adjust the temperature, and some organizations have two incubators, one set at each temperature range.

18.2-10 For how long are the samples incubated?

It depends on the process used. If one sample is incubated at two different temperatures, at least 7 days is required. See Box 5 in Section 6.2.2 of <797>[3] for detailed information.

18.2-11 What are the action levels for active air sampling?

The levels are different for each ISO classified area. See **Exhibit 18-1**.

EXHIBIT 18-1. Action Levels for Microbial Air Sampling

ISO Class	Action Level per Plate
5	More than 1 CFU per cubic meter of air
7	More than 10 CFU per cubic meter of air
8	More than 100 CFU per cubic meter of air

CFU = colony-forming unit

18.3 SURFACE SAMPLING

18.3-1 What does *surface sampling* mean?

Surface sampling means sampling the surfaces exposed to sterile compounding with a plate containing growth media. Any microbial contamination will be captured on the plate, which is then incubated.

18.3-2 What device is used for surface sampling?

For flat surfaces, use a contact plate. It has a convex surface that extends above the lip of the plate. For surfaces that are not flat (such as junctures of surfaces, equipment, etc.), a swab can be used.

18.3-3 What is measured by surface sampling?

Microbial contamination on the surfaces.

18.3-4 How often is surface sampling required?

Initially to established baseline levels of quality and to be sure the area is in a state of control. Then, monthly for Category 1 and 2; weekly for Category 3. Category 3 also requires additional testing following batches and self-enclosed robots. If growth above the action level is found, you will need to sample after remediation to be sure whatever caused the excursion has been corrected.

18.3-5 What surfaces have to be sampled?

All ISO-classified surfaces and pass-through chambers opening into classified areas must be sampled. The PEC deck (surface), the equipment in a PEC (such as a repeater pump, automated compounding device, workflow hardware, etc.), staging areas near the PEC (such as carts or counters), and frequently touched surfaces (such as counters, carts, pass-throughs, refrigerator handles, etc.) need to be included in the plan.

18.3-6 Do areas in the segregated compounding area (SCA) or containment segregated compounding area (C-SCA) have to be tested?

The PEC does. Consider testing areas within the perimeter of the PEC to be sure you are not compromising patient safety with contamination. However, testing the areas in the SCA or the C-SCA outside the PEC is not required by <797>. Note that you are likely to see growth, because the SCA or C-SCA does not have the controls of a cleanroom suite (such as ISO classification and HEPA-filtered ceiling air). Action levels are not applied to the samples collected in the SCA or C-SCA.

18.3-7 When is the sampling done?

At the end of compounding activities or end of shift but before the area has been cleaned and disinfected. Category 3 has additional requirements.

18.3-8 What areas are most likely to be at risk of contamination?

Surfaces where supplies are placed and other spots where activity occurs in the sterile compounding area are most likely to be at risk of contamination.

18.3-9 What media is used?

Use a general microbiological growth media (such as TSA) supplemented with additives (such as lecithin and polysorbate 80) that neutralize the effects of disinfecting agents. The plates or other devices used to sample flat surfaces must have a raised convex surface. For irregular surfaces, sterile swabs can be used which are then placed in or on the media. See Box 6 in Section 6.3.2 of <797>[3] for complete information.

18.3-10 Our laboratory doesn't stock the media listed in <797>. Can regular or blood agar plates be used?

No. You need to use a media that includes neutralizers so you won't get false negative results from residual disinfecting agents. Laboratory suppliers can provide the media you need.

18.3-11 What is the temperature required for incubators?

Two temperature ranges are required: 20–25 degrees C and 30–35 degrees C, so two incubators are needed.

18.3-12 For how long are the samples incubated?

It depends on the process used. If one sample is incubated at two different temperatures, at least 7 days is required. See Box 6 in Section 6.3.2 of <797>[3] for complete information.

18.3-13 Are plates required for surface sampling or are paddles OK?

Plates, paddles, or slides can be used. Plates are appropriate for flat surfaces. Swabs are appropriate for other surfaces; the sampling swab may need to be plated. Check the manufacturer's information and the details in <797>.

18.3-14 Is there a special type of plate to use for surface sampling?

Yes. Contact plates (i.e., RODAC™ [Replicate Organism Detection and Counting]) are used. They have a convex (not flat) surface.

18.3-15 Should I sample the same places each month or rotate areas?

Create a map of your sterile compounding area and mark the areas to test. You need to collect enough data to trend. Trended data should be evaluated at least annually and at that time, modifying sample locations may be appropriate based on the data.[52]

18.3-16 What are the action levels for surface sampling?

The levels are different for each ISO classified area. See **Exhibit 18-2.**

EXHIBIT 18-2. Action Levels for Surface Sampling

ISO Class	Action Level per Plate or Swab
5	More than 3 CFU
7	More than 5 CFU
8	More than 50 CFU

CFU = colony-forming unit

18.4 REACTING TO OUT-OF-SPECIFICATION RESULTS

18.4-1 What do I do when results are above the action level?

Action level excursions require you to look at the possible causes and attempt to remediate them.

18.4-2 Do I need to retest when out-of-specification results are found?

Yes. Once you have taken steps to remediate the issue, you need to retest to be sure the situation has been corrected.

18.4-3 There is 1 CFU of mold in the anteroom. What should I do?

Anterooms are the transition spaces between unclassified (not ISO classified) and controlled areas. It is not unusual to have some growth in the anteroom, even from mold. Even if the result is under the action level, you need to know that you have taken all appropriate steps to remediate what you can.

Some things to consider:

▶ Look at the location where the mold was found. Is it in the air or in a surface sample?

▶ Is this a repeated issue? If so, was the prior location the same?

▶ Is it near the sink?

▶ Is it near the entrance?

▶ Is it in or near a pass-through?

▶ Is it close to the refrigerator?

Determining sources can help you identify an appropriate remediation.

18.4-4 Where are likely sources of contamination?

Personnel, touch contamination, supplies, poor technique, work surfaces, and the air handling system are potential sources of contamination.

18.4-5 There is mold in the buffer room, but it's below the action level. What should I do?

Is this the first time you've found this or is it a frequent occurrence? Is it 1 CFU or always close to the action level? You need to evaluate the significance and frequency. Certainly, one immediate action is to check your cleaning practices and solutions. Be sure that you are using a sporicidal. Consider increasing the frequency of use of the sporicidal. Consider use weekly. If it is a negative pressure buffer room, be sure that the pressure is within the range of negative 0.010 to 0.030″ wc to adjacent space. A room that is too negative can pull in contamination from adjacent space (including the ceiling). Check your most recent certification report to be sure the integrity of the HEPA filters were recorded, and don't indicate a potential problem. Involve your infection control practitioner in the evaluation. Perhaps he or she has found similar contamination in other areas in your organization.

18.4-6 My hood is OK but my room isn't. What can I do until the room passes?

Unless there is an egregious situation in your SEC that you want to avoid using it or the PEC in it at all, you can consider this situation an SCA. You are then limited to Category 1 CSPs, including the limited BUD of 12 hours room temperature or 24 hours refrigerated. Your state board of pharmacy may have additional requirements.

18.4-7 What results do we have to report to our state board of pharmacy?

That depends on your state regulations. Be sure you are aware if and when you need to report excursions to the state board, other regulatory agency, or to a process defined in your policies and procedures.

QUALITY ASSURANCE AND QUALITY CONTROL *19*

19.1 What is the difference between quality control and quality assurance?

Quality control are the processes you check following compounding to be sure the compounded sterile preparation (CSP) is within the specifications you intend. It might include pH, color, specific testing, or other checks. *Quality assurance* is a system of processes developed so you can be sure the compounds meet the appropriate quality standards.

19.2 Does <797> define the characteristics I need to follow?

See *USP General Chapter <1163> Quality Assurance in Pharmaceutical Compounding*[53] for information on the elements you should include in your policies.

19.3 Are the components of a QA program limited to the CSPs?

They are related to the compounds but encompass more than that. For example, you need to be able to identify patient complaints, adverse drug reactions, and medication errors related to the CSPs. The designated person needs to oversee the system to be sure it complies with your policies and procedures, could detect problems, and appropriately addresses issues.[54]

19.4 What kinds of elements should we include on the report we present at the Infection Control Committee meeting?

This depends on the scope of your committee. Summary information should be reported to the appropriate committee (e.g., Infection Control, Quality, Pharmacy and Therapeutics). Be sure to report at the frequency defined in policy. Include those intervals when all results were within range considered acceptable (not just when issues are found).

Consider the following items in your report:

▶ Certification results, such as the status of the PECs and SECs (i.e., passed, failed, needs attention)

▶ Summary results of daily facility monitoring (e.g., number of days with acceptable readings, action taken for out of specification results)

▶ Number of personnel oriented to sterile compounding

▶ Personnel testing results (e.g., 9 out of 10 tests were within acceptable limits; 1 person was retested and waiting for results)

DOI 10.37573/9781585287260.019

▶ Results of environmental monitoring (e.g., number of samples taken and per-centage of results within acceptable limits, action taken on samples above the action level)

19.5   What are considered insanitary conditions?

The Food and Drug Administration (FDA) document *Insanitary Conditions at Compounding Facilities*[34] details the type of excursions considered unsanitary.

They include the following:

▶ Insects or rodents observed in or near compounding areas

▶ Visible contamination (both microbial and nonmicrobial)

▶ Handling different types of drugs without adequate separation to avoid cross-contamination

▶ Poor aseptic practices

▶ Storing open sterile containers without protective covers

▶ Use of nonsterile or nondepyrogenated containers or closures for sterile compounding

▶ Improper design or maintenance of the sterile compounding facility

▶ Insufficient sterilization time

▶ Use of improper filters

▶ Poor cleaning processes

Be sure your QA program addresses all of these issues.

WHAT DO I DO NOW? 20

20.1 I'm overwhelmed with this information. Where do I start?

▶ Read <797> and the FAQs on the USP site. There are also sterile compounding components in <800> and <825>.

▶ Perform a gap analysis. Compare the requirements (*must* statements) and recommendations (*should* and may statements) in <797> with your current practices.

▶ Assign a designated person and provide needed resources (e.g., educational programs).

▶ Attend in-person or online training sessions.

▶ Examine your certification report, discuss noncompliant issues with your certifier, and take steps to become compliant. Identify the facility issues you need to improve and obtain administrative approval for any renovations needed.

▶ Work with your designated person to ensure personnel training and policy development.

▶ Ensure your policies and procedures are appropriate.

▶ Be sure key individuals at your organization—the person to whom you report, the risk manager, others as appropriate—are aware of noncompliant issues for which you need resources.

▶ Network with other sterile compounding professionals.

20.2 Is there a template action plan I could use to start assessing the compliance at my organization?

Exhibit 20-1 is an example of an action plan.

DOI 10.37573/9781585287260.020

EXHIBIT 20-1. Example Action Plan for Compliance with USP <797>

	Element	Assigned To	Completed
List of CSPs			
Designated person			
Personnel training			
Garb	Gloves		
	Gowns		
	Other components		
Receiving	Training		
	Assess integrity of packages		
	Spill kit		
Sterile components and supply storage area			
Sterile compounding area			
Cleaning			
Quality assurance plan			

CSPs = compounded sterile preparations

FUTURE EDITIONS

Do you have questions that were not answered? Feel free to submit questions that can be included in the next edition of this publication. Send the questions to publications@ashp.org.

DOI 10.37573/9781585287260.FE

REFERENCES

1. United States Pharmacopeial Convention. Compounding Compendium. Rockville, MD: United States Pharmacopeia. *USP-NF 2023*, Issue 1, November 1, 2022.

2. United States Pharmacopeial Convention. General chapter <795> pharmaceutical compounding—nonsterile preparations. *USP-NF 2023*, Issue 1, November 1, 2022.

3. United States Pharmacopeial Convention. General chapter <797> pharmaceutical compounding—sterile preparations. *USP-NF 2023*, Issue 1, November 1, 2022.

4. United States Pharmacopeial Convention. General chapter <800> hazardous drugs—handling in healthcare settings. *USP-NF 2023*, Issue 1, November 1, 2022, official as of July 1, 2020.

5. United States Pharmacopeial Convention. General chapter <825> radiopharmaceuticals—preparation, compounding, dispensing, and repackaging. *USP-NF 2023*, Issue 1, November 1, 2022, official as of December 1, 2020.

6. Myers CE. History of sterile compounding in US hospitals: learning from the tragic lessons of the past. *Am J Health-Syst Pharm*. 2013;70:1414–1427.

7. Newton DW. United States Pharmacopeia chapter <797> timeline 1989 to 2013. *Int J Pharm Compd*. 2013;17:283-8.

8. United States Food and Drug Administration. Repackaging of certain human drug products by pharmacies and outsourcing facilities, 2017. https://www.fda.gov/downloads/Drugs/ Guidances/UCM434174.pdf. Accessed November 1, 2022.

9. Kienle PC. *The Chapter <800> Answer Book*. Bethesda, MD: ASHP, 2017.

10. United States Pharmacopeial Convention. General chapter <1168> compounding for phase 1 investigational studies. *USP-NF 2023*, Issue 1, November 1, 2022, official as of March 1, 2019.

11. United States Food and Drug Administration. Compounded drug products that are essentially copies of a commercially available drug product under section 503a of the federal Food, Drug, and Cosmetic Act guidance for industry, 2018. www.fda.gov/downloads/ Drugs/GuidanceComplianceRegulatoryInformation/Guidances/UCM510154.pdf. Accessed November 1, 2022.

12. ASHP Compounded Sterile Preparations Certificate for Pharmacists, 2021. https://elearning .ashp.org/products/9299/compounded-sterile-preparations-certificate-for-pharmacists. Accessed December 21, 2022.

13. Price AS, Meleis L, Childs C, et al. Access the resource impact of USP revisions. *Pharm Purch and Products*. 2022 (Jan): 8–12.

14. Board of Pharmacy Specialties. BPS Board Certified Sterile Compounding Pharmacist (BCSCP). www.bpsweb.org. Accessed November 1, 2022.

15. Pharmacy Technician Certification Board. Certified Compounded Sterile Preparation Technician Program. www.ptcb.org/about-ptcb/news-room/whats-new-at-ptcb/2017 /12/06/ptcb-launches-certified-compounded-sterile-preparation-technician-(cspt-) -program. Accessed November 1, 2022.

16. Murdaugh LB. *Competence Assessment Tools for Health-System Pharmacies*. 5th ed. Bethesda, MD: ASHP; 2015.

17. *Pharmacy Competency Assessment Center*. Bethesda, MD: ASHP; 2023.

18. United States Department of Labor. Occupational Safety and Health Administration. Hazard communication. https://www.osha.gov/dsg/hazcom/HCSFinalRegTxt.html. Accessed November 1, 2022.

DOI 10.37573/9781585287260.REF

19. Centers for Disease and Control Prevention. NIOSH list of antineoplastic and other hazardous drugs in healthcare settings, 2016. Publication number 2016-161. https://www.cdc.gov/niosh/docs/2016-161/pdfs/2016-161.pdf. Accessed November 1, 2022.

20. United States Department of Labor. Occupational Safety and Health Administration. Hazard communication: small entity compliance guide for employers that use hazardous chemicals. https://www.osha.gov/Publications/OSHA3695.pdf. Accessed November 1, 2022.

21. Centers for Disease Control and Prevention. Hand hygiene in healthcare settings. https://www.cdc.gov/handhygiene. Accessed November 1, 2022.

22. ASTM International. ASTM D6978 standard practice for assessment of resistance of medical gloves to permeation by chemotherapy drugs. https://www.astm.org/Standards/D6978.htm. Accessed November 1, 2022.

23. ASTM F739-12e1. Standard Test Method for Permeation of Liquids and Gases through Protective Clothing Materials under Conditions of Continuous Contact. West Conshohocken, PA: ASTM International. https://www.astm.org/standards/F739.htm. Accessed November 1, 2022.

24. Centers for Disease Control and Prevention. National Institute for Occupational Safety and Health. The national personal protective technology laboratory, respirator trusted-source information. https://www.cdc.gov/niosh/npptl/topics/respirators/disp_part/respsource.html. Accessed November 1, 2022.

25. Centers for Disease Control and Prevention. Safe injection practices to prevent transmission of infections to patients. https://www.cdc.gov/injectionsafety/ip07_standardprecaution.html. Accessed November 1, 2022.

26. Association for Professionals in Infection Control and Epidemiology. APIC position paper: safe injection, infusion, and medication vial practices in health care, 2016. https://www.apic.org/Resource_/TinyMceFileManager/Position_Statements/2016APICSIPPosition Paper.pdf. Accessed November 1, 2022.

27. Davis J, Ayars C. Retention of sterile compounding knowledge among pharmacy technicians. *J Pharm Technology*. 2021;1–6.

28. Buchanan C, Schneider P, Forrey R. *Compounding Sterile Preparations*. 4th ed. Bethesda, MD: ASHP; 2017.

29. United States Pharmacopeial Convention. General chapter <71> sterility tests. *USP-NF 2023*, Issue 1, November 1, 2022, official prior to 2013.

30. United States Food and Drug Administration. FD&C Act provisions that apply to human drug compounding. https://www.fda.gov/Drugs/GuidanceComplianceRegulatory Information/PharmacyCompounding/ucm606955.htm. Accessed November 1, 2022.

31. United States Pharmacopeial Convention. General chapter <1231> water for pharmaceutical purposes. *USP-NF 2023*, Issue 1, November 1, 2022, official as of December 1, 2021.

32. Controlled Environment Testing Association. CETA application guides. https://www.cetainternational.org/current-cags. Accessed November 1, 2022.

33. Institute for Safe Medication Practices. Guidelines for sterile compounding and the safe use of sterile compounding technology. https://www.ismp.org/resources/guidelines-sterile-compounding-and-safe-use-sterile-compounding-technology. Accessed November 1, 2022.

34. United States Food and Drug Administration. Insanitary conditions at compounding facilities, November 2020. https://www.fda.gov/media/124948/download. Accessed November 1, 2022.

35. United States Pharmacopeial Convention. General chapter <659> packaging and storage requirements. *USP-NF 2023*, Issue 1, November 1, 2022, official as of April 1, 2021.

36. Rhoads R, Exner L, Wagner JT. Demystifying dynamic smoke pattern tests for sterile compounding pharmacies. *Am J Health-Syst Pharm*. 2020;77:56-60.

37. Gianturco SL, Mattingly AN. Distinguishing between compounding facilities and the development of the 503B bulk drug substance list. *J Am Pharm Assoc.* 2021;Jan-Feb 61(1):e8-e11.

38. United States Food and Drug Administration. Bulk drug substances used in compounding under section 503a of the FD&C Act. **https://www.fda.gov/Drugs/GuidanceCompliance RegulatoryInformation/PharmacyCompounding/ucm614204.htm**. Accessed November 1, 2022.

39. United States Food and Drug Administration. Regulatory policy information. **https://www .fda.gov/drugs/human-drug-compounding/regulatory-policy-information**. Accessed November 1, 2022.

40. United States Pharmacopeial Convention. General chapter <1178> good repackaging practices. *USP-NF 2023*, Issue 1, November 1, 2022, official as of December 1, 2020.

41. American Society of Health-System Pharmacists. ASHP guidelines on compounding sterile preparations. *Am J Health-Syst Pharm.* 2014;71:145-66.

42. Power LA, Coyne JW. ASHP guidelines on handling hazardous drugs. *Am J Health-Syst Pharm.* 2018;75:1996-2031.

43. Centers for Disease Control and Prevention. Biosafety in microbiological and biomedical laboratories (BMBL). 6th ed. **www.cdc.gov/labs/BMBL.html**. Accessed November 1, 2022.

44. International Journal of Pharmaceutical Compounding. **www.ijpc.com**. Accessed November 1, 2022.

45. Centers for Disease Control and Prevention. Guidelines for the prevention of intravascular catheter-related infections. **www.cdc.gov/mmwr/preview/mmwrhtml/mm5132a9.htm**. Accessed November 1, 2022.

46. American Society of Health-System Pharmacists. *ASHP Injectable Drug Information 2023.* Bethesda, MD: ASHP; 2023.

47. Simpson MC, Schaefer EG, *Extended Stability for Parenteral Drugs.* 7th ed. Bethesda, MD: ASHP; 2023.

48. King Guide Publications, Inc. *King Guide to Parenteral Admixtures.* Napa, CA: King Guide Publications; 2019. **https://kingguide.net**. Accessed November 1, 2022.

49. United States Food and Drug Administration. MedWatch: the FDA safety information and adverse event reporting program. **https://www.fda.gov/safety/medwatch-fda-safety -information-and-adverse-event-reporting-program**. Accessed November 1, 2022.

50. Rutala WA, Weber DJ. Selection of the ideal disinfectant. *Inf Control and Hosp Epidemiology.* 2014;35:855–863.

51. United States Pharmacopeial Convention. General chapter <1113> microbial characterization, identification, and strain typing. *USP-NF 2023*, Issue 1, November 1, 2022, official prior to 2013.

52. Tharp JC, Kullar RK, Tupps MA. Designing a microbiological monitoring program for compounding facilities. *Am J Health-Syst Pharm.* 2021;78:158–167.

53. United States Pharmacopeial Convention. General chapter <1163> quality assurance in pharmaceutical compounding. *USP-NF 2023*, Issue 1, November 1, 2022, official as of December 1, 2020.

54. Janusziewicz AN, Glueck SN, Park SY, et al. A pharmacist-driven Food and Drug Administration incident surveillance and response program for compounded drugs. *Am J Health-Syst Pharm.* 2021;78:1438–1443.

INDEX

A

accreditation organizations, 1

action levels, 6
- for air sampling, 135–136
- gloved fingertip and thumb test and, 48
- in sampling plan, 132
- for surface sampling, 138, 139–140

action plan, 143–144

active air sampling, 134–136

active pharmaceutical ingredients (APIs)
- beyond-use dates (BUDs) of, 112
- compounding, 97
- eye and respiratory risk when working with, 27
- use of, 55–56

addEASE®, 95, 112

ADD-Vantage™, 95, 112

administration of medications, 37–41
- administration, defined, 37
- compounding distinguished from, 11
- policies concerning, 37
- preparation for, 37–38

air changes per hour (ACPH)
- for air handing system, 73
- calculating, 68
- for chemo room, 67
- for cleanroom suite, 73
- for containment segregated compounding area, 75
- facility requirements for, 59, 62–63
- for IV room, 66
- for segregated compounding area, 63
- for storage room, 64

air flow
- dwell time and, 120
- dynamic air flow testing of PEC, 84
- environmental monitoring and, 131
- in pass-through chambers, 72, 77, 78
- training and, 41

air handling system, 62, 66, 85, 139

albumin, 98

alcohol as disinfectant/sanitizing agent, 120, 126

alcohol-based hand sanitizer, 28

alert level, 132

algorithm, 95–96

allergenic extracts, 5, 7
- compounding area, 80–81
- compounding process, 101
- immediate use and, 40

allergenic extracts compounding area (AECA), 69, 80–81

amber dropper bottles, 97

American Chemical Society (ACS) marking, 56

anesthesia personnel, 40

animals, application of USP <797> to, 9

anterooms, 68–71
- active air sampling in, 135
- air changes per hour (ACPH) in, 59, 62
- cleaning, 70, 128
- in cleanroom suite, 66, 70–71, 72–73, 74, 75
- dirty side distinguished between clean side, 70
- facility requirements for, 68–71
- garb and, 28, 30–31, 34
- gloved fingertip and thumb test in, 47, 48
- line of demarcation in, 68, 70
- mold in, 139
- office space in, cleaning, 128
- pass-through chambers to, 76
- pressure in, 66, 67, 69, 72, 85

antibiotics
- beyond-use-dates, 113
- master formulation record (MFR) for, 100
- saline bag used for reconstituting, 113
- syringes, reconstituted and frozen, 110
- vials, reconstitution of, 38

Aseptic Compounding Technique: Learning and Mastering the Ritual, 42

aseptic technique, 5, 50
- beyond-use dates (BUDs) and, 105, 106
- competency in, 15, 41
- immediate use preparations and, 11
- insanitary conditions and, 142
- training in, 50

ASTM F739-12e1 (*Standard Test Method for Permeation of Liquids and Gases through Protective Clothing Materials under Conditions of Continuous Contact*), 30

ASTM Standard D6978, the *Standard Practice for Assessment of Resistance of Medical Gloves to Permeation by Chemotherapy Drugs*, 29–30

autoclaves, 41, 97, 105

autologous serum, 98